# Essential Skills for Medical Social Work

# Essential Skills for Medical Social Work

## A Guide to Competence, Compassion, and Clinical Impact


Dr. Kenshara Cravens-Knoxson, LMSW, CCM, LCDC (CI)

*Prairie View A&M University*



cognella
SAN DIEGO

Bassim Hamadeh, CEO and Publisher
Amy Smith, Associate Editorial Manager
Dani Nouriazad, Associate Production Editor
Emely Villavicencio, Senior Graphic Designer
Brianna Lucas, Licensing Coordinator
Tiffany Mok, Senior Content Marketing Specialist
Natalie Piccotti, Director of Marketing
Kassie Graves, Senior Vice President, Editorial
Alia Bales, Director of Project Editorial & Production



Printed in the United States of America.

# Contents

# Disclaimer

Note: Portions of this book were developed with the assistance of ChatGPT, a language model created by OpenAI, to help organize ideas, generate drafts, and refine content. All content has been reviewed and edited for accuracy and relevance by the author.

OpenAI. (2024). *ChatGPT* (Mar 14 version) [Large language model]. https://chat.openai.com/

# Acknowledgments

This book emerges from lived experience, dedicated practice, and the steadfast belief that social work, particularly in health care settings, represents both a professional calling and a refined craft.

To the patients and families who granted me access to the most intimate moments of their lives: Thank you. Your resilience, vulnerability, and trust have profoundly shaped my professional identity. I carry your stories with care and honor.

To my colleagues in nursing, medicine, chaplaincy, therapy, case management, and especially fellow social workers, your collaboration, wisdom, and humor have sustained me through the most complex clinical situations. You have reminded me repeatedly that this work is never accomplished in isolation.

To my mentors and supervisors, thank you for creating spaces for reflection, growth, and advocacy. You taught me that ethical practice often requires courage over convenience, and that presence frequently holds more healing power than intervention.

To the next generation of medical social workers, I wrote this book for you. May it serve as a guide, a mirror, and a reminder that your work matters more than you may ever fully comprehend. The profession needs your voice, your compassion, and your commitment to justice.

Finally, to my family and loved ones, thank you for the patience, encouragement, and grace that allowed me to write through work, life, and everything between. Your belief in me is woven into every page.

With deep gratitude,
Dr. Kenshara Cravens-Knoxson

# Introduction

## The Critical Role of Medical Social Work in Contemporary Health Care

Medical social work plays a crucial role in health care. Medical social workers connect clinical expertise, system navigation, and human advocacy to bridge the gap between medical treatment and the psychosocial factors that impact health outcomes (Beder, 2006; Gehlert & Browne, 2012). While physicians diagnose and treat disease, and nurses provide direct care and monitoring, social workers attend to the human dimensions of illness: the fear, the grief, the financial strain, the family conflict, and the systemic barriers that shape whether a patient can actually follow through with a treatment plan.

Despite this critical role, many social workers enter medical settings feeling underprepared for the specific demands of health care environments. Graduate social work education, while comprehensive in theory and generalist practice, often provides limited exposure to the rapid pace, medical terminology, interdisciplinary dynamics, and life-and-death stakes that characterize hospital and clinical practice (Cowles & Lefcowitz, 1992; Dziegielewski, 2013). New practitioners may find themselves navigating complex discharge planning processes, facilitating end-of-life conversations, or responding to acute crises with minimal preparation for these specialized interventions.

This gap between academic preparation and practice reality motivated the creation of this book. Drawing from both empirical research and practice wisdom accumulated over years of direct clinical experience, this text aims to bridge the divide between what social workers learn in graduate programs and what they need to know to practice effectively and ethically in medical settings.

## The Evolution of Medical Social Work

Medical social work has evolved significantly since its origins in the early 20th century, when pioneers like Ida Cannon established social work departments in hospitals to address the social and environmental factors affecting patient health (Beder, 2006). What began as a focus on connecting patients with community resources and addressing environmental health hazards has expanded into a sophisticated practice that encompasses crisis intervention, complex discharge planning, ethics consultation, advance care planning, and systems advocacy (Gehlert & Browne, 2012).

Contemporary medical social workers practice across diverse settings including acute care hospitals, rehabilitation facilities, outpatient clinics, hospice and palliative care programs, and integrated behavioral health environments. In each of these contexts, social workers contribute specialized expertise in psychosocial assessment, care coordination, patient and family counseling, and navigation of health care and community service systems (National Association of Social Workers [NASW], 2016).

Research consistently demonstrates that social work interventions improve patient outcomes, reduce hospital readmissions, enhance patient and family satisfaction, and address health disparities (Coulton et al., 1982; Jack et al., 2009). Yet social work contributions often remain undervalued or misunderstood within health care organizations, where biomedical models of care may overshadow the psychosocial dimensions of health and healing (Dziegielewski, 2013).

## Evidence-Based Practice in Medical Social Work

This book is grounded in the principles of evidence-based practice, which integrates the best available research evidence with clinical expertise and patient values to guide intervention decisions (Rubin & Parrish, 2012). Throughout the following chapters, you will find theoretical frameworks, empirical research findings, and practice guidelines that support the recommendations and strategies presented.

However, evidence-based practice in social work extends beyond the application of research findings. It also encompasses practice-based evidence, the systematic documentation and analysis of what works in real-world clinical encounters (Epstein, 2011). This book honors both forms of knowledge, putting together research literature with case examples, practical strategies, and reflection questions designed to deepen your clinical reasoning and professional judgment.

## Organization and Use of This Book

The 25 chapters that follow are organized into five thematic sections, each addressing essential competencies for effective medical social work practice:

**Section 1: Clinical Foundations** establishes the fundamental knowledge base required for medical social work practice, including medical terminology, health care systems navigation, common health conditions, psychosocial assessment, and trauma-informed care. These foundational competencies enable social workers to communicate effectively with interdisciplinary colleagues, understand the medical context of patients' lives, and conduct thorough biopsychosocial assessments.

**Section 2: The Heart of Patient and Family Care** explores the relational and supportive dimensions of social work practice, including crisis intervention, grief and loss support, cultural competence, discharge planning, and advance care planning. These chapters emphasize the centrality of the therapeutic relationship and the art of being present with patients and families during vulnerable moments.

**Section 3: Ethics, Advocacy, and Equity** addresses the ethical foundations and social justice imperatives that guide medical social work practice. Chapters in this section cover patient rights and autonomy, mandated reporting obligations, ethical decision-making frameworks, health equity, and relevant health care laws and policies. This section affirms the social worker's role as an advocate and ethical anchor within health care teams.

**Section 4: Teamwork and System Navigation** focuses on collaborative practice and systems thinking, essential skills for effectiveness in complex health care organizations. Topics include interprofessional communication, care coordination across settings, clinical documentation, community resource development, and conflict navigation. These competencies enable social workers to function as valuable team members and skilled system navigators.

**Section 5: Growth and Leadership in Social Work** addresses professional sustainability and development, including self-care and burnout prevention, licensure and supervision, cultural humility, mentorship, and staying current in an evolving field. These chapters recognize that effective practice requires ongoing attention to professional growth and personal well-being.

Each chapter follows a consistent structure designed to facilitate learning and application:

1. **Learning objectives** identify the key competencies addressed in the chapter
2. **Literature reviews** provide theoretical foundations and research context
3. **Main content** integrates evidence-based knowledge with practical application
4. **Practical tips** offer concrete strategies grounded in research and practice wisdom
5. **Reflection questions** encourage critical thinking and self-examination
6. **Key takeaways** summarize essential points for quick reference

This structure supports multiple uses of the book. Graduate students may read it sequentially to build comprehensive knowledge. New practitioners might focus on specific chapters addressing immediate practice challenges. Experienced social workers may use it as a reference text or for continuing education. Field instructors and supervisors can utilize the reflection questions and case studies to structure learning conversations with students and supervisees.

## Who This Book Is For

This book is written primarily for three audiences:

- **Graduate social work students** preparing for field placements or careers in health care settings will find comprehensive preparation for medical social work practice. The book addresses topics often underemphasized in generalist MSW curricula while connecting specialized practice to core social work values and theories.
- **New and early-career medical social workers** navigating the transition from graduate education to professional practice will discover practical guidance for common challenges, from conducting rapid psychosocial assessments to navigating interdisciplinary team dynamics to managing the emotional demands of health care practice.
- **Experienced medical social workers** seeking to deepen their practice or transition to new health care settings will benefit from the integration of current research, evidence-based frameworks, and opportunities for reflective practice. The book can support continuing education requirements, preparation for clinical licensure, or specialized certification.

Field instructors, supervisors, and social work educators may also find this text valuable for structuring learning experiences, facilitating supervision conversations, and teaching specialized content in medical social work courses.

## A Note on Terminology and Inclusivity

Throughout this book, I use “patient” to refer to individuals receiving health care services, recognizing that some settings and professionals prefer “client,” “resident,” or “member.” I use “social worker” to encompass both master’s level and licensed clinical social workers, specifying level of licensure only when relevant to scope of practice discussions.

I have made every effort to use inclusive language that honors the diversity of patients, families, and colleagues we serve. When discussing cultural considerations, I aim to avoid essentializing or stereotyping while acknowledging that culture profoundly shapes health beliefs, family structures, and care preferences. I encourage readers to approach all generalizations with critical thinking, recognizing that individual variation within any cultural group exceeds differences between groups.

## The Way Forward

Medical social work is challenging work. It demands clinical knowledge, emotional presence, ethical clarity, cultural humility, systems thinking, and personal resilience. You will encounter heartbreak and hope, often in the same shift. You will witness suffering you cannot eliminate and face systemic barriers you cannot singlehandedly dismantle. You will question whether your interventions make sufficient difference.

Social work in health care is truly impactful. You will support families facing tough decisions and guide them toward choices that reflect their values. You will link isolated elders to services that help them stay in their homes. You will advocate for patients whose voices often go unheard. You will simplify complex medical information with compassion. You will be there during important moments when your presence makes a significant difference.

This book cannot prepare you for every situation you will encounter. Health care is too complex, human suffering too varied, and each patient's story too unique for any single text to anticipate all possibilities. What this book can offer is a framework for thinking about your practice, a foundation of evidence-based knowledge, and the reassurance that the questions and struggles you experience are shared by social workers across settings and career stages.

As you read the chapters that follow, I encourage you to engage actively with the material. Reflect on the questions posed. Consider how the research and frameworks apply to your specific practice context. Notice your emotional responses to difficult topics. Seek supervision or consultation when material raises unresolved issues. Use this book as a starting point for deeper learning, not as a final authority.

The profession of social work needs your voice, your passion, and your commitment to both clinical excellence and social justice. Health care needs social workers who can hold complexity, bear witness to suffering, and persistently advocate for human dignity within systems that too often prioritize efficiency over compassion.

Welcome to this essential work. May this book support your journey toward competence, compassion, and enduring clinical impact.

## References

Beder, J. (2006). *Hospital social work: The interface of medicine and caring*. Routledge.

Coulton, C. J., Dunkle, R. E., Goode, R. A., & MacKintosh, J. (1982). Discharge planning and decision making. *Health & Social Work, 7*(4), 253–261. https://doi.org/10.1093/hsw/7.4.253

Cowles, L. A., & Lefcowitz, M. J. (1992). Interdisciplinary expectations of the medical social worker in the hospital setting. *Health & Social Work, 17*(1), 57–65. https://doi.org/10.1093/hsw/17.1.57

Dziegielewski, S. F. (2013). *The changing face of health care social work: Opportunities and challenges for professional practice* (3rd ed.). Springer Publishing Company.

Epstein, I. (2011). Reconciling evidence-based practice, evidence-informed practice, and practice-based research: The role of clinical data-mining. *Social Work, 56*(3), 284–288. https://doi.org/10.1093/sw/56.3.284

Gehlert, S., & Browne, T. (Eds.). (2012). *Handbook of health social work* (2nd ed.). John Wiley & Sons.

Jack, B. W., Chetty, V. K., Anthony, D., Greenwald, J. L., Sanchez, G. M., Johnson, A. E., Forsythe, S. R., O'Donnell, J. K., Paasche-Orlow, M. K., Manasseh, C., Martin, S., & Culpepper, L. (2009). A reengineered hospital discharge program to decrease rehospitalization: A randomized trial. *Annals of Internal Medicine, 150*(3), 178–187. https://doi.org/10.7326/0003-4819-150-3-200902030-00007

National Association of Social Workers. (2016). *NASW standards for social work practice in health care settings*. NASW Press.

Rubin, A., & Parrish, D. E. (2012). Outcomes of social work intervention with older adults: A systematic review. *Journal of Evidence-Based Social Work, 9*(1–2), 88–107. https://doi.org/10.1080/15433714.2012.636329

Section I

# Clinical Foundations

Before you can effectively advocate, counsel, or coordinate care, you need a strong clinical foundation. In medical social work, clinical expertise extends beyond diagnosing mental health conditions to encompass understanding health care systems, medical language, and the psychosocial impact of illness and treatment. This section establishes the groundwork for everything that follows.

The five chapters in this section will help you develop essential competencies:

- **Speaking the language** of healthcare professionals and translating it for patients
- **Navigating complex systems** and understanding organizational structures
- **Recognizing common medical conditions** and their psychosocial implications
- **Conducting comprehensive psychosocial assessments** that inform interventions
- **Practicing trauma-informed care** in every clinical interaction

These skills position you as a trusted member of the care team, someone who can communicate across disciplines, support patients through crisis, and bridge the gap between biomedical treatment and holistic healing. The chapters that follow provide both theoretical foundations and practical strategies to strengthen your clinical practice in medical settings.

CHAPTER 1

# Understanding Medical Terminology

## Learning Objectives

By the end of this chapter, you will be able to do the following:

- Recognize and appropriately use essential medical terminology in healthcare settings
- Translate complex medical language into patient-friendly explanations
- Communicate effectively with interdisciplinary team members using shared clinical vocabulary
- Build strategies for continuous learning of medical terminology

## The Critical Role of Medical Language in Social Work Practice

Language serves as currency in healthcare settings. The ability to understand and appropriately use medical terminology directly influences your effectiveness as a social worker, your credibility with colleagues, and your capacity to advocate for patients (Reeves et al., 2017). When physicians, nurses, and case managers discuss patient care using clinical shorthand, social workers must comprehend not only the words themselves but also their implications for psychosocial functioning and discharge planning.

Medical terminology fluency enables social workers to participate meaningfully in interdisciplinary rounds, understand documentation in electronic health records, and identify critical details that shape intervention planning (Bronstein, 2003). Without this foundation, social workers risk missing essential information, misinterpreting treatment goals, or delaying necessary psychosocial interventions.

Consider a scenario in which the medical team describes a patient experiencing "CHF exacerbation." A social worker unfamiliar with this terminology might not immediately recognize that congestive heart failure is worsening, potentially missing the urgency of addressing home safety, medication access, and caregiver support before discharge. Understanding that "exacerbation" signals deterioration rather than stability fundamentally changes the discharge planning conversation.

The translation function represents an equally important dimension of medical terminology competence. Patients and families frequently feel overwhelmed by medical jargon, struggling to comprehend diagnoses, treatment plans, and prognoses (Berkman et al., 2011). Social workers serve as interpreters, converting complex clinical language into accessible explanations that support informed decision-making. This bridging role requires both understanding the medical terminology and possessing the communication skills to explain concepts clearly without condescension or oversimplification.

Research on interprofessional collaboration consistently identifies shared language as a foundation for effective teamwork (D'Amour et al., 2005). When social workers demonstrate medical knowledge through appropriate terminology use, other healthcare professionals more readily recognize social work expertise and value social workers' contributions to care planning. Conversely, unfamiliarity with basic medical terms can undermine professional credibility and marginalize social work voices in team discussions.

## Essential Medical Terminology for Social Work Practice

The following terminology represents foundational knowledge for medical social workers across practice settings. While exhaustive memorization proves neither necessary nor realistic, familiarity with these common terms enables more effective practice and provides a framework for continued learning.

**Table 1.1** Patient Status and Cognitive Function

| Term | Definition | Practice Implications |
|---|---|---|
| A&O x3 or x4 | Alert and Oriented to person, place, time, and sometimes situation | Provides baseline information for capacity assessment and safety planning |
| LOC | Level of Consciousness | Changes may indicate delirium, medication effects, or neurological changes requiring immediate attention |
| Capacity | Clinical determination of ability to understand and make healthcare decisions | Differs from legal competency; social workers often participate in capacity assessments |

**Table 1.2** Common Medical Conditions

| Term | Definition | Psychosocial Considerations |
|---|---|---|
| ARDS | Acute Respiratory Distress Syndrome | Severe lung condition requiring intensive care; family crisis intervention needs |
| CABG | Coronary Artery Bypass Graft | Major heart surgery requiring significant recovery; lifestyle modifications needed |
| C. diff | *Clostridioides difficile* infection | Contagious intestinal infection; isolation precautions affect family visitation |
| CHF | Congestive Heart Failure | Chronic condition with frequent exacerbations; discharge planning complexity |

| Term | Definition | Psychosocial Considerations |
|---|---|---|
| COPD | Chronic Obstructive Pulmonary Disease | Progressive condition affecting breathing; home oxygen and mobility considerations |
| DVT | Deep Vein Thrombosis | Blood clot risk; may require anticoagulation and activity restrictions |
| ESRD | End-Stage Renal Disease | Requires dialysis; significant treatment burden and quality of life impacts |
| FTT | Failure to Thrive | Concerning decline, especially in elderly or children; may trigger APS/CPS involvement |
| Sepsis | Life-threatening response to infection | Medical emergency; family crisis support needs |
| TIA | Transient Ischemic Attack | "Mini-stroke" warning sign; urgent need for prevention strategies |

**Table 1.3** Medical Procedures and Interventions

| Term | Definition | Social Work Relevance |
|---|---|---|
| BKA | Below Knee Amputation | Significant functional change; grief, adaptation, and prosthetic access needs |
| Foley | Urinary catheter | Requires care assistance; impacts discharge planning for home |
| G-tube/PEG tube | Gastrostomy/feeding tube | Long-term nutritional support; caregiver training and home care coordination |
| NPO | Nothing by mouth (*nil per os*) | Patient cannot eat or drink; may cause distress requiring explanation |

| Term | Definition | Social Work Relevance |
|---|---|---|
| TPN | Total Parenteral Nutrition | IV nutrition for patients unable to use GI tract; complex home care needs |
| Vent/Ventilator | Mechanical breathing support | Intensive care requirement; advance directive discussions often needed |
| Wound Vac | Negative pressure wound therapy | Specialized wound care; impacts placement options and home care |

**Table 1.4** Clinical Settings and Team Communications

| Term | Definition | Practice Application |
|---|---|---|
| Code Status | Resuscitation preferences (Full Code, DNR, etc.) | Central to advance care planning and goals of care discussions |
| H&P | History and Physical examination | Initial comprehensive assessment documenting medical status |
| I&O | Intake and Output monitoring | Fluid balance tracking; important for renal and cardiac patients |
| RRT | Rapid Response Team | Activated for acute patient deterioration; crisis intervention may follow |
| Stat | Immediately (*statim*) | Indicates urgency; prioritization needed |
| Telemetry | Continuous cardiac monitoring unit | Higher acuity setting; family education about monitoring equipment |

## Strategies for Building Medical Terminology Competence

Developing medical terminology fluency represents an ongoing process rather than a finite achievement. The following evidence-based strategies support continuous learning:

1. **Create a personal medical glossary.** Maintain a digital or written compilation of unfamiliar terms encountered in practice. Recording definitions, contexts of use, and implications for social work practice strengthens retention and creates a personalized reference tool (Bogo, 2015). Review and expand this glossary regularly, particularly when transitioning to new practice settings or patient populations.
2. **Engage in active translation practice.** After hearing medical terminology in team meetings or documentation, practice explaining the concept in plain language. This exercise strengthens both comprehension and communication skills essential for patient education and advocacy (Berkman et al., 2011). Consider partnering with a colleague for mutual translation practice.
3. **Request clarification without hesitation.** Asking for explanation of unfamiliar terms demonstrates professional humility and commitment to thorough understanding rather than ignorance (Tervalon & Murray-García, 1998). Frame questions constructively: "Can you help me understand what you mean by..." or "I want to make sure I'm explaining this correctly to the family. When you say...."
4. **Review documentation systematically.** Electronic health records contain extensive medical terminology in physician notes, nursing assessments, and diagnostic reports. Allocate time to review these documents carefully, looking up unfamiliar terms and observing how clinicians describe patient conditions and treatment plans (Reamer, 2013).
5. **Utilize reputable medical references.** Several high-quality resources support medical terminology learning:
   - *MedlinePlus Medical Dictionary* (National Library of Medicine)
   - *Mosby's Medical Dictionary* for healthcare professionals
   - Specialty-specific glossaries from professional organizations
   - Hospital orientation materials and approved abbreviation lists
6. **Participate actively in interdisciplinary rounds.** Regular exposure to team discussions provides contextual learning opportunities. Listen attentively to how team members use terminology, noting connections between medical language and treatment decisions (Bronstein, 2003).

## Practical Application: The Art of Translation

Understanding medical terminology proves insufficient without the ability to translate this knowledge into accessible patient communication. Health literacy research demonstrates that many patients struggle to comprehend medical information, leading to poor adherence, confusion about treatment, and difficulty participating in shared decision-making (Berkman et al., 2011).

Effective translation involves several key principles:

1. **Use plain language consistently.** Replace medical jargon with everyday words: *serious infection* instead of *sepsis*; *heart attack* instead of *myocardial infarction*; and *bone break* instead of *fracture*. The teach-back method, asking patients to explain information in their own words, verifies understanding (Agency for Healthcare Research and Quality [AHRQ], 2015).
2. **Provide context and relevance.** Connect medical information to patient concerns and daily life: "Your heart isn't pumping as strongly as it should, which is why you've been feeling so tired and short of breath."
3. **Check for understanding regularly.** Avoid asking "Do you understand?" which often prompts affirmative responses regardless of actual comprehension. Instead, use open-ended questions: "What questions do you have about this?" or "How would you explain this to your family?"
4. **Account for cultural and linguistic differences.** When working with interpreters, speak directly to the patient while allowing adequate time for interpretation. Recognize that some medical concepts may not translate directly across languages or cultural frameworks (Sue & Sue, 2016).

## Critical Thinking Questions

1. Analyze the relationship between medical terminology fluency and professional power dynamics within interdisciplinary healthcare teams. How does language competence influence the perceived value of social work contributions to patient care?
2. From a health equity perspective, examine how medical jargon creates barriers to patient understanding and informed consent. What theoretical frameworks help explain the relationship between health literacy, language accessibility, and health disparities?
3. Critically evaluate the tension between developing biomedical knowledge and maintaining social work's distinct biopsychosocial perspective. How can social workers integrate medical fluency without adopting reductionist biomedical frameworks?
4. Consider the ethical implications of translation work in healthcare settings. What responsibilities do social workers bear when serving as interpreters of medical information, and how does this role intersect with principles of patient autonomy and self-determination?

## Key Takeaways

- Medical terminology fluency enables effective interdisciplinary communication and strengthens professional credibility.
- Social workers serve a critical translation function, converting medical jargon into accessible patient education.
- Understanding medical language directly impacts assessment quality, discharge planning effectiveness, and patient advocacy.
- Continuous learning strategies include maintaining a personal glossary, requesting clarification, and reviewing documentation systematically.
- Plain language communication and teach-back methods verify patient understanding and support informed decision-making.

CHAPTER 2

# Navigating Health Systems

## Learning Objectives

By the end of this chapter, you will be able to do the following:

- Identify key organizational structures and processes within health care systems
- Distinguish between various health care settings and levels of care
- Recognize roles and responsibilities of interdisciplinary team members
- Navigate institutional policies and procedures effectively
- Understand payor systems and their influence on care access

## Understanding Health Care System Complexity

Health care delivery in the United States operates through various organizations, regulations, payment mechanisms, and professional roles. This complexity creates significant challenges for patients attempting to access care and for professionals working to coordinate services across settings (Burau & Blank, 2006). Medical social workers function as essential navigators within this complex system, requiring comprehensive understanding of organizational structures, care pathways, and institutional processes.

Research demonstrates that system navigation represents a core social work competency, directly influencing patient outcomes, care continuity, and resource utilization (McDonald et al., 2007). Social workers who thoroughly understand health care systems can anticipate barriers, expedite necessary services, and advocate effectively when institutional policies conflict with patient needs. On the other hand, insufficient system knowledge contributes to delayed discharges, fragmented care, and missed opportunities for intervention.

The ability to navigate health care systems encompasses multiple dimensions: understanding organizational hierarchies and decision-making processes, recognizing how different settings serve distinct patient populations, knowing how payment sources shape service availability, and identifying the appropriate channels for addressing problems or concerns (Dziegielewski, 2013). This systems literacy enables social workers to function as effective advocates and care coordinators rather than being overwhelmed or stymied by institutional complexity.

### Health Care Settings and Levels of Care

Medical social workers practice across a continuum of care settings, each with distinct purposes, patient populations, regulatory requirements, and professional norms. Understanding these differences proves essential for appropriate service coordination and discharge planning.

**Acute care hospitals** provide short-term medical treatment for serious conditions, injuries, or surgical procedures. These fast-paced environments emphasize rapid assessment, stabilization, and transition to lower levels of care. Social workers in acute care settings typically carry high caseloads, conduct brief psychosocial assessments, facilitate discharge planning, and respond to crises. Length of stay pressures influence practice patterns, requiring efficient intervention and documentation (Dziegielewski, 2013).

**Long-term acute care hospitals (LTACHs)** serve medically complex patients requiring extended hospitalization beyond typical acute care stays, often involving ventilator weaning, wound care, or recovery from severe illness. Social workers address prolonged hospitalization impacts on patients and families, coordinate complex discharge plans, and facilitate goals of care discussions when prognosis remains uncertain.

**Inpatient rehabilitation facilities (IRFs)** provide intensive therapy services for patients recovering from strokes, traumatic injuries, amputations, or major surgeries. These settings require patients to participate in at least three hours of therapy daily. Social workers coordinate family training, address adjustment to disability, and plan for community reintegration with necessary supports and equipment.

**Skilled nursing facilities (SNFs)** offer 24-hour nursing care and rehabilitation services, serving both short-term recovery and long-term care needs. Medicare-covered short-term stays require specific documentation of skilled needs and improvement potential. Social workers navigate complex regulatory requirements while addressing psychosocial adjustment, family dynamics, and potential transitions to other settings.

**Outpatient clinics** deliver ongoing care for chronic conditions, preventive services, and specialty treatments. Social work roles vary widely, from integrated behavioral health to disease-specific education and support. These settings allow for relationship development over time and focus on self-management support and community resource connection.

**Hospice and palliative care programs** serve patients with serious or terminal illnesses, focusing on comfort, quality of life, and family support. Hospice specifically serves patients with prognoses of six months or less. Social workers provide grief counseling, advance care planning facilitation, practical support, and bereavement services. These settings demand comfort with death, grief, and existential concerns (Kramer et al., 2013).

**Home health care** brings medical and supportive services into patients' homes, serving homebound individuals requiring skilled nursing or therapy. Social workers assess home environments, address safety concerns, coordinate equipment and services, and support caregivers managing complex care responsibilities.

## The Interdisciplinary Health Care Team

Effective practice within health care systems requires understanding the roles, responsibilities, and perspectives of various team members. While terminology and specific role definitions vary across institutions, core team members typically include:

**Physicians and advanced practice providers** lead medical diagnosis and treatment planning. Attending physicians hold ultimate responsibility for patient care, while residents and fellows participate in teaching hospitals. Nurse practitioners and physician assistants provide direct care and may serve as primary providers in some settings. Understanding medical hierarchy and decision-making authority helps social workers identify appropriate contacts for specific concerns.

**Registered nurses (RNs)** coordinate direct patient care, administer medications, monitor patient status, and serve as frontline communicators with physicians. Nurses often possess detailed knowledge of patient responses to treatment, family dynamics, and emerging concerns. Charge nurses manage unit operations and can facilitate problem-solving when issues arise.

**Case managers** focus primarily on utilization review, insurance authorization, and discharge logistics. While case management and social work roles overlap in some institutions, many hospitals maintain separate departments. Understanding these distinctions prevents duplication and facilitates collaboration. Case managers typically possess detailed knowledge of insurance requirements and placement processes (Powell Davies et al., 2008).

**Physical, occupational, and speech therapists** assess functional abilities and rehabilitation potential. Physical therapists address mobility and ambulation. Occupational therapists focus on activities of daily living and adaptive equipment. Speech-language pathologists evaluate swallowing safety and communication abilities. Therapy recommendations significantly influence discharge planning and placement decisions.

**Pharmacists** manage medication safety, identify drug interactions, and counsel patients about medication use. Clinical pharmacists participate in rounds and provide consultation on complex medication regimens, which is particularly valuable for patients with multiple chronic conditions.

**Chaplains and spiritual care providers** address spiritual and existential concerns, provide ritual support, and facilitate meaning-making during illness and loss. Collaboration with chaplains strengthens whole-person care and prevents social workers from carrying sole responsibility for spiritual support.

**Care coordination and navigation programs** employ various titles (patient navigators, care coordinators, community health workers) for professionals who help patients access services, understand health information, and overcome barriers to care. These roles complement social work and present collaboration opportunities.

Understanding how these roles interact and where responsibilities overlap or diverge enables social workers to leverage team expertise effectively while clarifying their unique contributions (Bronstein, 2003).

## Critical Institutional Processes

Several key processes structure health care delivery and directly impact social work practice:

1. **Interdisciplinary rounds** convene team members to review patient status, treatment plans, and discharge readiness. Rounds may occur at bedsides or in conference rooms. Social workers who participate actively in rounds, presenting relevant psychosocial information concisely, strengthen their team integration and influence care planning (Reeves et al., 2017).
2. **Utilization review** evaluates whether hospital stays and services meet medical necessity criteria established by payors. Utilization review nurses or case managers track length of stay against expected benchmarks and work to prevent insurance denials. Social workers must understand these processes to anticipate discharge pressure and advocate when psychosocial factors necessitate continued hospitalization.
3. **Discharge planning** ideally begins at admission and involves progressive assessment of post-hospital needs, family resources, and service coordination. Effective discharge planning requires early identification of barriers, proactive communication with patients and families, and collaboration across disciplines (Shepperd et al., 2013). Many institutions implement formal discharge planning protocols and screening tools.
4. **Care transitions and handoffs** involve transferring patient care responsibility between providers, teams, or settings. Poor communication during transitions contributes to medical errors and adverse events. Social workers facilitate effective transitions by providing comprehensive psychosocial summaries, warm handoffs to community providers, and follow-up coordination (Coleman et al., 2006).

## Payor Systems and Their Influence

Payment mechanisms profoundly shape service availability, length of stay, and discharge options. While social workers are not billing specialists, basic understanding of payor systems proves essential for realistic planning and patient advocacy.

**Medicare** provides federal insurance for individuals aged 65 and older and certain younger people with disabilities. Medicare Part A covers hospital stays and skilled nursing facility care under specific conditions. Part B addresses outpatient services and physician fees. Part D covers prescription medications. Understanding Medicare coverage rules, particularly the three-day hospital stay requirement for SNF coverage and homebound status for home health, informs discharge planning.

**Medicaid** offers state-administered insurance for low-income individuals and families. Medicaid eligibility and benefits vary significantly by state. Many nursing home residents rely on Medicaid after depleting private resources. Medicaid often covers services not included in Medicare, such as long-term care and transportation.

**Private insurance** encompasses diverse plans with varying coverage rules, networks, and authorization requirements. Managed care plans may restrict provider choice and require pre-authorization for services. High-deductible plans create significant out-of-pocket costs that influence patient decisions and adherence.

**Uninsured and self-pay patients** face significant barriers to care access and post-acute services. Social workers advocate for charity care programs, pharmaceutical assistance, and community resources. Financial counselors collaborate with social work to address insurance enrollment and payment arrangements.

Understanding payor limitations enables realistic discharge planning while identifying where advocacy might expand options. Documentation of medical necessity for services, particularly when psychosocial factors complicate care, can influence coverage decisions.

### Navigating Institutional Barriers

Health care systems contain inherent tensions between efficiency and quality, cost containment and comprehensive care, institutional priorities and patient needs. Social workers frequently encounter situations where policies or processes conflict with optimal patient care. Effective navigation requires:

1. **Building strategic relationships** with key contacts across departments strengthens your ability to solve problems and access resources. Discharge planners, financial counselors, ethics committee members, and patient advocates become valuable collaborators.
2. **Understanding formal channels** for addressing concerns or challenging decisions (ethics consultations, patient advocacy offices, formal appeal processes) provides appropriate escalation pathways when needed.
3. **Documenting thoroughly** creates a record of barriers encountered, advocacy efforts undertaken, and rationales for recommendations. Clear documentation protects both patients and practitioners while supporting quality improvement efforts.
4. **Balancing advocacy and pragmatism** acknowledges that while systems contain flaws and injustices, working effectively within existing structures often achieves better immediate outcomes for patients than confrontational approaches. Strategic advocacy chooses battles carefully while maintaining commitment to systemic change.

## Critical Thinking Questions

1. Apply organizational theory to analyze health care system complexity. How do bureaucratic structures, professional hierarchies, and institutional policies shape social work practice and patient experiences?
2. Compare and contrast the Medicare and Medicaid systems from a social justice perspective. How do payment structures perpetuate or mitigate health disparities, and what advocacy strategies might address systemic inequities?
3. Examine the concept of "medical necessity" as socially constructed rather than objectively defined. How do utilization review processes reflect particular values and priorities, and what populations are most disadvantaged by these determinations?
4. Critically analyze the role of social workers as system navigators. Does this function primarily

serve to help individuals adapt to unjust systems, or does it create opportunities for systemic change? Support your position with theoretical frameworks.

## Key Takeaways

- Health care system complexity requires social workers to understand organizational structures, care settings, and institutional processes.
- Different care settings (e.g., acute hospitals, rehabilitation, skilled nursing, home health, hospice) serve distinct purposes and populations.
- Effective interdisciplinary collaboration depends on understanding team member roles and leveraging collective expertise.
- Payor systems significantly influence service availability and discharge planning options.
- Strategic relationship-building and thorough documentation strengthen system navigation effectiveness.

CHAPTER 3

# Common Health Conditions and Comorbidities

## Learning Objectives

By the end of this chapter, you will be able to do the following:

- Recognize common health conditions encountered in medical social work practice
- Understand the psychosocial implications of various medical diagnoses
- Identify patterns of comorbidity and their impact on patient functioning
- Apply biopsychosocial assessment to medical conditions
- Anticipate social work needs based on diagnosis and disease trajectory

## The Biopsychosocial Framework in Medical Social Work

Medical social workers operate at the intersection of biological, psychological, and social dimensions of health and illness. The biopsychosocial model, first articulated by George Engel (1977), revolutionized medical understanding by challenging purely biomedical conceptualizations of disease. This framework recognizes that biological pathology does not exist in isolation but interacts dynamically with psychological factors (thoughts, emotions, behaviors) and social contexts (relationships, culture, environment, socioeconomic status) to shape health experiences and outcomes (Borrell-Carrió et al., 2004).

For social workers in health care settings, the biopsychosocial model provides both a conceptual framework for understanding illness and a practical tool for comprehensive assessment and intervention. While physicians focus primarily on biological pathology and treatment, social workers attend to how illness affects functioning, relationships, identity, and quality of life. This attention to the full human experience of illness distinguishes social work's contribution to patient care.

Research consistently demonstrates that psychosocial factors profoundly influence health outcomes, treatment adherence, symptom management, and recovery (Katon, 2011). Depression, for instance, complicates diabetes management, increases cardiovascular risk, and contributes to poor surgical outcomes. Social isolation accelerates cognitive decline in dementia and increases rehospitalization risk for heart failure patients. Financial strain creates barriers to medication adherence and follow-up care across all conditions.

Understanding common medical conditions and their typical psychosocial implications enables social workers to conduct targeted assessments, anticipate challenges, and coordinate appropriate interventions. While each patient's experience remains unique, patterns emerge across diagnostic categories that inform practice.

# Common Medical Conditions in Social Work Practice

The following conditions represent those most frequently encountered across medical social work settings. Understanding their basic pathophysiology, treatment approaches, and common psychosocial impacts strengthens assessment and intervention planning.

## Cardiovascular Conditions

**Congestive heart failure (CHF)** occurs when the heart cannot pump blood effectively, causing fluid accumulation in lungs and extremities. Patients experience fatigue, shortness of breath, and activity intolerance that significantly limit function (Hunt et al., 2009). Psychosocial considerations include

- depression and anxiety related to activity limitations and uncertain prognosis
- complex medication regimens requiring cognitive capacity and financial resources
- dietary restrictions (sodium, fluid) that may conflict with cultural food practices
- frequent hospitalizations that disrupt employment, relationships, and independence
- end-of-life planning needs given progressive disease course

**Stroke (cerebrovascular accident)** causes sudden brain damage due to interrupted blood flow, resulting in varying degrees of paralysis, speech impairment, cognitive changes, and functional loss. The abrupt nature of disability creates crisis for patients and families (Stroke Unit Trialists' Collaboration, 2013). Social workers address

- acute grief over lost abilities and changed identity
- caregiver burden and relationship strain
- depression affecting rehabilitation participation and recovery
- discharge planning complexity based on functional abilities
- long-term disability planning including financial and legal needs

## Pulmonary Conditions

**Chronic obstructive pulmonary disease (COPD)** encompasses chronic bronchitis and emphysema, progressive conditions that impair breathing. Most cases result from smoking, sometimes creating stigma and blame (Global Initiative for Chronic Obstructive Lung Disease, 2023). Psychosocial dimensions include

- anxiety and panic related to breathlessness
- social isolation due to oxygen dependence and activity limitations
- depression complicating disease management
- smoking cessation support needs
- home safety assessment for oxygen use
- advance care planning given progressive deterioration

## Endocrine Conditions

**Diabetes mellitus** affects the body's ability to produce or use insulin and requires ongoing management through diet, medication, and monitoring. Both Type 1 and Type 2 diabetes carry significant self-management burden and complication risk (American Diabetes Association, 2023). Social workers address

- health literacy needs for complex self-management
- financial barriers to medication, supplies, and diabetic-appropriate food
- depression and diabetes distress affecting adherence

- family dynamics and cultural beliefs about diet
- complication management including vision loss, neuropathy, and amputation adjustment

## Neurological Conditions

**Dementia and Alzheimer's disease** involve progressive cognitive decline affecting memory, judgment, and functional independence. Patients and families face prolonged illness trajectory with mounting care needs (Alzheimer's Association, 2023). Social work interventions include

- safety assessment and caregiver support
- advance care planning while patient retains capacity
- connection to respite services and support groups
- behavioral management strategies
- long-term care planning and financial counseling
- grief support for patient and family

## Oncology

**Cancer** encompasses diverse diseases with varying prognoses and treatment demands. Social work needs vary based on cancer type, stage, treatment plan, and prognosis (National Comprehensive Cancer Network, 2023). Common psychosocial concerns include

- fear of death and existential distress
- treatment decision-making support
- side effect management affecting quality of life
- financial toxicity from treatment costs
- body image concerns and relationship impacts
- advance care planning and hospice transitions
- survivorship adjustment and fear of recurrence

## Renal Conditions

**End-stage renal disease (ESRD)** requires dialysis or transplantation for survival. The treatment burden significantly affects quality of life and functioning (United States Renal Data System, 2023). Social workers address

- emotional impact of chronic, demanding treatment
- transportation to dialysis sessions
- dietary and fluid restrictions
- employment and disability planning
- transplant evaluation and waitlist support
- advance care planning including dialysis withdrawal

## Mental Health and Substance Use Disorders

Mental health diagnoses and substance use disorders frequently co-occur with medical conditions and complicate treatment (Katon, 2011). Social workers provide

- integrated behavioral health interventions
- connection to psychiatric treatment and substance use services
- medication adherence support
- relapse prevention planning

- stigma reduction through education and advocacy
- treatment of co-occurring conditions affecting medical recovery

### Chronic Pain

Chronic pain affects physical functioning, mental health, relationships, and quality of life. The opioid epidemic has complicated pain management, creating additional stigma and barriers (Institute of Medicine, 2011). Social work interventions include

- psychosocial pain assessment
- connection to multidisciplinary pain management
- support for functional goal setting
- assistance with disability applications
- addressing isolation and depression
- coordination with pain management and behavioral health services

## Understanding Comorbidities

Comorbidity refers to the presence of multiple health conditions simultaneously. Comorbidity patterns are not random; certain conditions cluster together due to shared risk factors, pathophysiological connections, or treatment side effects (Valderas et al., 2009). For example,

- diabetes, hypertension, and heart disease frequently co-occur
- COPD and heart failure often appear together
- chronic pain commonly presents with depression and anxiety
- substance use disorders complicate virtually all medical conditions

Comorbidities exponentially increase complexity across multiple dimensions (Vogeli et al., 2007):

1. **Medical complexity:** Multiple conditions require more medications, specialist appointments, and treatment coordination. Medications for one condition may complicate another. Symptoms from different conditions overlap, making assessment challenging.
2. **Self-management burden:** Patients juggle competing treatment demands, dietary restrictions, and medication schedules. Cognitive load increases while capacity may decrease due to age or illness.
3. **Psychosocial stress:** Multiple diagnoses create cumulative emotional impact. Financial strain multiplies with each condition. Functional limitations compound, affecting independence and quality of life.
4. **Health care navigation challenges:** Patients see multiple specialists who may not coordinate care. Fragmented systems create gaps and duplications. Insurance coverage varies across conditions and providers.

Social workers play a critical role in helping patients and families navigate comorbidity complexity. Interventions include care coordination, prioritization assistance, system navigation, and advocacy for integrated rather than fragmented care approaches.

## Diagnosis and Discharge Planning

Understanding medical diagnoses and their typical trajectories informs discharge planning and intervention timing. Consider the following.

1. **Progressive vs. acute conditions:** Progressive conditions like dementia or COPD require anticipatory planning and periodic reassessment as functioning declines. Acute conditions like stroke or hip fracture focus on recovery maximization and adjustment to potentially permanent changes.
2. **Rehabilitation potential:** Some conditions (stroke, orthopedic surgery) carry strong rehabilitation potential, influencing appropriateness of intensive rehabilitation settings. Others (advanced dementia, end-stage cancer) focus on comfort and function maintenance.
3. **Permanence of changes:** Temporary functional limitations suggest different planning than permanent disability. Adjustment counseling, equipment needs, and caregiver training vary accordingly.
4. **Prognosis and time course:** Terminal diagnoses raise hospice eligibility and advance care planning urgency. Chronic conditions with years-long trajectories allow gradual planning and periodic intervention.
5. **Treatment intensity and side effects:** Aggressive cancer treatment may temporarily worsen function before improvement. Medications may cause cognitive dulling, fatigue, or other symptoms affecting daily life.

# Practical Application: Assessment Questions

Effective assessment connects medical diagnosis to lived experience. Rather than focusing solely on medical facts, ask questions.

- "How has this condition affected your daily life?"
- "What worries you most about living with this diagnosis?"
- "What has been hardest for your family?"
- "How are you managing the treatment demands?"
- "What makes it harder or easier to follow your treatment plan?"
- "How is this condition affecting your work, relationships, or activities you value?"

These questions reveal the psychosocial dimensions of illness that medical assessments may miss but that fundamentally shape coping, adherence, and outcomes.

# Critical Thinking Questions

1. Evaluate the biopsychosocial model's strengths and limitations in contemporary health care practice. What aspects of human experience might this framework inadequately address, and what complementary theoretical perspectives could strengthen holistic understanding?
2. Analyze comorbidity through the lens of social determinants of health. How do structural factors (poverty, racism, environmental conditions) contribute to clustering of multiple chronic conditions, and what implications does this have for intervention design?
3. Consider the medicalization of social problems and its implications for social work practice. How do diagnostic categories shape our understanding of patient experiences, and when might medical framing obscure social and structural contributors to suffering?
4. Examine the concept of "patient education" critically. How do assumptions about health literacy and compliance reflect particular cultural values and power relations? What alternative frameworks might better support equitable health promotion?

## Key Takeaways

- The biopsychosocial model provides a framework for understanding how biological, psychological, and social factors interact to shape health experiences.
- Common medical conditions carry predictable psychosocial implications that inform social work assessment and intervention.
- Comorbidities exponentially increase complexity in medical management, self-care burden, and psychosocial stress.
- Understanding disease trajectories and prognoses enables appropriate discharge planning and intervention timing.
- Assessment questions should explore how illness affects daily life, relationships, and functioning rather than focus solely on medical facts.

CHAPTER 4

# Conducting Psychosocial Assessments

## Learning Objectives

By the end of this chapter, you will be able to do the following:

- Conduct comprehensive psychosocial assessments in medical settings
- Apply standardized assessment frameworks and tools appropriately
- Distinguish assessment priorities in acute vs. ongoing care settings
- Integrate cultural responsiveness into assessment processes
- Document assessment findings clearly and professionally

## The Centrality of Assessment in Social Work Practice

Psychosocial assessment represents the foundation of effective social work intervention, the process through which social workers gather information, identify needs, understand strengths, and develop intervention plans (Hepworth et al., 2016). In medical settings, where interventions often must occur rapidly and within narrow time constraints, assessment quality directly influences appropriateness and effectiveness of services provided.

Unlike medical assessment focused on diagnosis and treatment of disease, psychosocial assessment explores how illness, hospitalization, and treatment affect the whole person within their life context (Jordan & Franklin, 2011). This holistic perspective distinguishes social work's contribution to patient care and positions social workers to identify needs invisible to other team members focused on biomedical dimensions.

Research demonstrates that thorough psychosocial assessment improves care planning, enhances patient satisfaction, identifies safety concerns, and reduces readmission risk (Bywaters & McLeod, 1996). Conversely, inadequate assessment leads to inappropriate discharge plans, missed opportunities for intervention, and potential harm when risks go unrecognized.

In medical settings characterized by rapid patient turnover and competing demands, assessment often must occur efficiently while remaining thorough enough to inform clinical decisions. This tension requires social workers to develop skills in rapid rapport-building, focused inquiry, and integration of information from multiple sources.

# Fundamental Domains of Psychosocial Assessment

Comprehensive psychosocial assessment explores multiple dimensions of patient experience and functioning. While specific assessment tools and institutional documentation forms vary, core domains remain consistent across settings (NASW, 2016).

**Mental health and emotional functioning** encompass current mood, anxiety, cognitive status, coping patterns, and psychiatric history. Observe for signs of depression (flat affect, psychomotor retardation, expressed hopelessness), anxiety (restlessness, worried expression, difficulty concentrating), or cognitive impairment (orientation deficits, memory problems, difficulty following conversation). Screen for suicidal ideation when depression or hopelessness emerge, using direct questions: "Have you had thoughts of hurting yourself or ending your life?" Inquire about previous mental health diagnoses, treatment, and current psychiatric medication use (Jordan & Franklin, 2011).

**Substance use history** addresses current and past alcohol and drug use, including prescription medication misuse. Substance use disorders frequently complicate medical treatment, affect surgical outcomes, create withdrawal risks during hospitalization, and influence discharge safety (Saitz, 2014). Normalize questions about substance use: "Many people use alcohol or other substances to cope with stress or pain. Can you tell me about your use?" Assess quantity, frequency, last use, and previous treatment attempts. Note that hospitalization may trigger withdrawal symptoms requiring medical management.

**Social support systems** evaluate the quality and availability of relationships that provide emotional support, practical assistance, and connection. Identify who the patient lives with, who visits during hospitalization, who helps with health management, and the quality of these relationships. Absence of support signals high-risk discharge, while strained relationships may complicate care planning (Cohen, 2004).

Explore:

"Who do you rely on when you need help?"

"How do family members feel about your illness?"

"Are there conflicts about your care?"

**Living situation and housing stability** assesses home safety, accessibility, and stability. Document number of floors, presence of stairs, bathroom safety features, home maintenance adequacy, and neighborhood safety. Housing instability or homelessness profoundly complicates discharge planning and health management (Berkowitz et al., 2013).

Screen for housing concerns:

"Do you have safe, stable housing?"

"Are you worried about being able to return home?"

"What challenges do you face at home?"

**Financial resources and employment status** influences access to medications, medical equipment, follow-up care, and basic needs. Assess income sources (employment, disability benefits, retirement, family support), insurance coverage, and out-of-pocket health care costs. Financial strain creates significant barriers to care adherence and contributes to medication non-adherence and missed appointments (Sommers & Singh, 2021). Many patients experience embarrassment discussing financial struggles; normalize these inquiries: "Medical costs create stress for many people. How are you managing the financial impact of your illness?"

**Cultural and spiritual beliefs** shape health understanding, decision-making, coping, and family roles. Inquire about cultural background, primary language, health beliefs, spiritual or religious practices, and preferences for decision-making involvement. Avoid assumptions based on perceived ethnicity or cultural markers. Ask open-ended questions: "What's important to me to understand about your cultural background?" "How do your beliefs influence how you make health decisions?" (Sue & Sue, 2016)

**Legal and safety concerns** include guardianship, power of attorney, custody issues, domestic violence, elder or child abuse, and criminal justice involvement. Document existing advance directives and identify legal surrogate decision-makers if capacity is questionable. Screen for abuse with direct, private questions: "Do you feel safe at home?" "Has anyone hurt you or threatened you?" Mandatory reporting obligations apply when abuse or neglect is suspected (Mathews & Bross, 2008).

**Functional status and caregiving needs** evaluates ability to perform activities of daily living (ADLs: bathing, dressing, toileting, eating, transferring) and instrumental activities of daily living (IADLs: medication management, meal preparation, financial management, transportation). Functional limitations directly influence discharge planning and service needs. Assess both current hospital functioning and baseline pre-illness status, as hospitalization often temporarily reduces function (Granger et al., 1998).

## Assessment in Acute Care Settings

Assessment in acute hospital settings presents unique challenges including brief patient encounters, high acuity and medical complexity, family crisis and emotional volatility, and pressure for rapid discharge planning. These constraints require social workers to prioritize assessment domains, gather information efficiently, and integrate data from multiple sources (Dziegielewski, 2013).

**Rapid rapport building** enables patients to share sensitive information quickly. Strategies include the following.

- Clear introduction of name, role, and purpose: "I'm the social worker. My role is to help with challenges illness creates beyond the medical treatment."
- Expressing empathy and normalizing distress: "Being in the hospital is stressful. Many people feel overwhelmed."
- Asking permission: "Is now an okay time to talk?"

  "Would you prefer if family stayed or if we spoke privately?"

- Active listening with minimal interruption
- Cultural responsiveness and use of professional interpreters when needed

**Focused Inquiry** prioritizes assessment areas most relevant to immediate needs rather than attempting exhaustive assessment. For a patient admitted for pneumonia with expected short stay, assessment might emphasize medication access, home safety for recovery, and support for ADLs. For a patient with new stroke and significant disability, comprehensive assessment of living situation, caregiver capacity, financial resources, and functional limitations becomes essential.

**Multi-source data integration** strengthens assessment accuracy. Sources include the following:

- direct patient interview and observation
- family or caregiver interview
- medical chart review (medical history, current medications, physician assessment)
- nursing observation of functional status and family dynamics
- therapy evaluations of mobility and self-care abilities
- previous social work documentation if patient known to system
- communication with outside providers or agencies

Information triangulation from multiple sources provides more complete and accurate understanding than relying solely on patient self-report, which may be limited by cognitive impairment, minimization, or insufficient insight.

## Standardized Assessment Tools

Validated assessment instruments strengthen assessment reliability and facilitate communication across disciplines. Listed here are some common tools in medical social work:

1. **Patient Health Questionnaire-9 (PHQ-9)** screens for depression severity using nine items corresponding to DSM diagnostic criteria. Scores guide clinical decision-making about psychiatric referral and intervention intensity (Kroenke et al., 2001).
2. **Generalized Anxiety Disorder-7 (GAD-7)** assesses anxiety symptom severity through seven items. This brief screen identifies patients requiring anxiety treatment (Spitzer et al., 2006).
3. **CAGE Questionnaire** provides a quick substance use screen using four items addressing attempts to Cut down, Annoyance at criticism, Guilt about use, and need for Eye-opener drinks. Positive screens warrant more thorough substance use assessment (Ewing, 1984).
4. **Confusion Assessment Method (CAM)** detects delirium, an acute confusional state common in hospitalized elders. Delirium indicates medical urgency and affects capacity assessment (Inouye et al., 1990).
5. **Mini-Mental State Examination (MMSE)** offers cognitive screening, though copyright restrictions limit use in some settings. Montreal Cognitive Assessment (MoCA) provides an alternative (Folstein et al., 1975).

While standardized tools provide valuable data, they supplement rather than replace comprehensive clinical assessment. Cultural factors, literacy levels, and current medical status may affect tool validity. Interpret results within broader assessment context rather than relying solely on numerical scores.

## Cultural Responsiveness in Assessment

Assessment approaches must adapt to cultural differences in communication styles, family structures, health beliefs, and help-seeking patterns. Research demonstrates that culturally insensitive assessment leads to misdiagnosis, inappropriate intervention, and disengagement from services (Ortega & Faller, 2011).

**Avoid assumptions** based on perceived ethnicity, accent, or appearance. Individual variation within cultural groups exceeds differences between groups. Ask about background rather than assuming knowledge.

**Adjust communication styles** to match patient and family preferences. Some cultures emphasize indirect communication and require time to establish trust before disclosing personal information. Others value directness. Follow the patient's lead.

**Recognize diverse family structures** and decision-making patterns. In some cultures, family collectively makes decisions rather than individuals acting autonomously. Respect these patterns rather than imposing Western individualism (Sue & Sue, 2016).

**Address language barriers appropriately** through professional interpretation services. Never use family members, especially children, as interpreters for medical or psychosocial assessment. Speak directly to the patient while allowing adequate interpretation time. Avoid idioms or complex language that may not translate well.

**Explore health beliefs and practices** without judgment. Many patients utilize traditional healing alongside Western medicine. These practices may or may not conflict with medical treatment. Understanding beliefs enables collaborative rather than combative approaches.

## Documentation of Assessment Findings

Assessment documentation serves multiple purposes: communicating findings to the care team, establishing the need for social work services, creating a legal record, and supporting continuity of care. Effective documentation balances thoroughness with clarity and conciseness (Reamer, 2005).

**Include relevant assessment domains** without excessive detail. Document findings that inform intervention planning or discharge decisions. Omit tangential information.

**Use objective, professional language** avoiding judgment or bias. Describe observed behaviors rather than characterizing patients: "Patient tearful when discussing family conflict" rather than "Patient is a drama queen."

**Distinguish between patient report and social worker observation.** Use phrases such as "Patient reports..." or "Patient states..." for subjective information and "Social worker observed..." for your direct observations.

**Note sources of information** when incorporating data from family, medical records, or other providers: "Per daughter, patient requires assistance with all ADLs" or "Nursing staff report patient becomes agitated in evenings."

**Connect assessment to intervention plan** so readers understand clinical reasoning. Document how identified needs lead to specific referrals or interventions: "Given patient's limited mobility and absence of caregiver support, recommend skilled nursing facility placement for rehabilitation."

**Maintain confidentiality and HIPAA compliance** by including only information relevant to care. Remember patients can access their medical records; write with this in mind.

# Critical Thinking Questions

1. Examine psychosocial assessment through a critical theory lens. How do assessment processes reflect and potentially reinforce power imbalances between practitioners and patients? What alternative assessment approaches might center patient expertise and lived experience more fully?
2. Analyze the tension between standardized assessment tools and individualized clinical judgment. What are the benefits and risks of relying on quantitative measures in psychosocial assessment, and how might evidence-based practice principles guide appropriate integration?
3. Consider cultural assessment from a perspective of cultural humility rather than cultural competence. How do essentializing assumptions about cultural groups potentially harm individuals, and what assessment approaches avoid these pitfalls while remaining culturally responsive?
4. Evaluate the concept of "rapid assessment" in acute care settings. What critical information might be sacrificed in the interest of efficiency, and how do time constraints disproportionately affect certain patient populations? What organizational changes might better support thorough assessment?

# Key Takeaways

- Psychosocial assessment provides the foundation for all social work interventions and distinguishes social work's holistic perspective.
- Comprehensive assessment explores mental health, substance use, social support, housing, finances, culture, legal issues, and functional status.
- Acute care settings require focused assessment, rapid rapport-building, and integration of information from multiple sources.
- Standardized assessment tools supplement but do not replace comprehensive clinical assessment.
- Cultural responsiveness requires avoiding assumptions, adapting communication, and exploring health beliefs without judgment.

- Assessment documentation should be objective, relevant, source-attributed, and connected to intervention planning.

CHAPTER 5

# Practicing Trauma-Informed Care

## Learning Objectives

By the end of this chapter, you will be able to do the following:

- Define trauma-informed care and explain its relevance to medical settings
- Apply the six principles of trauma-informed care in practice
- Recognize trauma responses in patients and families
- Implement trauma-sensitive communication and intervention strategies
- Address vicarious trauma and secondary traumatic stress in practitioners

## Understanding Trauma and Its Impact

Trauma results from experiences that overwhelm an individual's capacity to cope, creating lasting effects on neurobiological, psychological, and social functioning (van der Kolk, 2014). Traumatic experiences include childhood abuse or neglect, domestic violence, sexual assault, combat exposure, serious accidents, natural disasters, sudden loss, and systemic oppression based on race, gender, or other identities. Medical events themselves, including life-threatening diagnoses, invasive procedures, prolonged hospitalization, and ICU experiences, can constitute trauma (Substance Abuse and Mental Health Services Administration [SAMHSA], 2014).

Research documents the prevalence and impact of trauma exposure. The Adverse Childhood Experiences (ACE) Study demonstrated that childhood trauma correlates with adult chronic diseases, mental illness, substance use disorders, and early mortality (Felitti et al., 1998). Approximately 61% of adults report at least one ACE, with trauma exposure particularly concentrated among marginalized populations experiencing systemic oppression and violence.

Trauma affects brain development and functioning, particularly in areas governing emotional regulation, threat perception, and stress response. Traumatized individuals may experience hypervigilance, emotional dysregulation, difficulty trusting others, dissociation, and exaggerated startle responses. These neurobiological changes are adaptive responses to danger that become maladaptive when they persist in safe environments (van der Kolk, 2014).

Health care settings can trigger trauma responses, particularly for individuals with histories of medical trauma, abuse, or loss of control. Aspects of medical care that may be re-traumatizing include

- physical restraint or forced treatment
- lack of privacy during examinations or care
- feeling unheard or dismissed by providers

- loss of autonomy and control
- painful or invasive procedures
- experiences of discrimination or disrespect
- separation from support systems

Trauma-informed care emerged from recognition that traditional health care and behavioral health approaches often inadvertently re-traumatized individuals, particularly those with histories of abuse, by replicating power dynamics and failing to recognize trauma's pervasive effects (Harris & Fallot, 2001). This framework fundamentally shifts from asking "What's wrong with you?" to "What happened to you?" recognizing that behaviors often labeled as "difficult," "noncompliant," or "manipulative" may represent trauma responses and survival strategies.

## The Six Principles of Trauma-Informed Care

SAMHSA (2014) articulated six principles that guide trauma-informed organizational practice. While initially developed for behavioral health settings, these principles apply equally to medical social work and health care more broadly.

**Safety** emphasizes creating physical and emotional safety for patients and staff. In practice, this includes

- ensuring privacy during sensitive conversations
- explaining procedures before initiating them
- minimizing coercive interventions
- addressing environmental factors (noise, lighting, crowding) that trigger distress
- respecting personal space and asking permission before touching
- creating predictable routines when possible

**Ask yourself** "Does this patient feel safe right now? What might make them feel unsafe, and how can I address those factors?"

**Trustworthiness and transparency** involve clear, consistent communication and keeping commitments. Trauma often involves betrayal and broken trust; rebuilding trust requires reliability. Practices include

- explaining your role and limits of confidentiality clearly
- following through on commitments and explaining when circumstances prevent this
- being honest about unknowns and limitations
- acknowledging mistakes and apologizing when appropriate
- providing clear information about processes and timelines

Avoid promising outcomes you cannot guarantee. If you say you will call at 2 p.m., call at 2 p.m. or explain why you cannot.

**Peer support** recognizes the healing power of connection with others who have faced similar challenges. In medical settings, this includes

- facilitating connections to patient support groups
- leveraging patient navigators or peer mentors when available
- encouraging family and friend involvement when desired by patient
- sharing stories of others who have coped with similar challenges (with permission and maintaining confidentiality)

**Collaboration and mutuality** minimize power differentials and recognize that healing happens in relationships characterized by respect and shared power. Implementation strategies include

- involving patients actively in care planning
- asking "What would be most helpful?" rather than telling patients what they need
- recognizing patients as experts on their own experiences
- acknowledging that your role is to support, not fix
- using collaborative language: "Let's figure this out together"

**Empowerment, voice, and choice** center patient autonomy and strengthen self-efficacy. In health care settings where patients often experience powerlessness, intentionally offering choices and respecting decisions proves especially important. This includes

- offering options when possible: "Would you prefer to talk now or later today?"
- respecting refusal while exploring concerns: "You don't have to answer that. Can you tell me what makes that question uncomfortable?"
- highlighting strengths: "You've managed really difficult situations before"
- supporting self-advocacy and informed decision-making
- believing patient accounts of their experiences

**Cultural, historical, and gender issues** require recognizing how cultural background, historical trauma, and identity-based oppression shape trauma experiences and healing. This includes

- understanding that communities of color, LGBTQ+ individuals, and other marginalized groups experience systemic trauma
- recognizing medical mistrust rooted in historical abuses (Tuskegee Syphilis Study, forced sterilization, etc.)
- adapting approaches based on cultural healing practices and preferences
- addressing discrimination and bias in current health care delivery
- using preferred names, pronouns, and culturally resonant communication

# Recognizing Trauma Responses in Medical Settings

Trauma manifests through diverse responses that may appear across physical, emotional, cognitive, and behavioral domains. Recognizing these presentations enables compassionate, appropriate responses rather than judgment or conflict (SAMHSA, 2014).

**Hyperarousal and hypervigilance** appear as exaggerated startle responses, constant scanning of environment, inability to relax, difficulty sleeping, irritability, or aggressive reactions to perceived threats. A patient who appears "paranoid" or "difficult" may be experiencing trauma-based hypervigilance.

**Dissociation and numbing** manifests as emotional flatness, appearing disconnected or "checked out," memory gaps, and difficulty maintaining conversation focus. Patients may seem "noncompliant" when, in actuality, they are dissociating from overwhelming experiences.

**Re-experiencing** includes flashbacks, nightmares, and intense distress when exposed to trauma reminders. Medical procedures may trigger flashbacks for abuse survivors. Patients may refuse care not from "noncompliance" but from overwhelming trauma activation.

**Avoidance** leads individuals to avoid people, places, conversations, or activities triggering trauma memories. This may appear as missed appointments, refusal of certain providers, or resistance to discussing specific topics.

**Negative changes in mood and cognition** encompass persistent fear, horror, anger, guilt, shame, diminished interest in activities, feeling detached from others, and inability to remember aspects of traumatic events. Depression and substance use often co-occur with trauma.

**Control-seeking behaviors** may emerge as attempts to establish safety through controlling interactions. Patients may make excessive demands, refuse to cooperate with plans, or insist on specific providers. These behaviors often represent trauma-based needs for control rather than personality disorders.

Understanding these responses prevents misattribution of trauma symptoms to personality pathology or willful noncompliance. Trauma-informed practice responds to these presentations with compassion and strategic intervention rather than frustration or punishment.

# Trauma-Informed Communication and Intervention

Integrating trauma-informed principles into daily practice requires intentional communication strategies and relationship approaches that promote safety, respect autonomy, and avoid re-traumatization (Bloom & Farragher, 2013).

**Universal trauma precautions** assume that everyone may have trauma history, eliminating the need to identify trauma before providing trauma-sensitive care. This approach prevents overlooking trauma in those who do not disclose and creates generally safer, more respectful care for all.

**Clear communication about roles and processes** reduces anxiety created by uncertainty. Begin interactions by introducing yourself, explaining your role, describing what will happen, and asking permission: "I'm Miriam, the social worker. My role is to help with challenges beyond medical treatment. I'd like to talk with you about your support at home and any concerns about discharge. Is now a good time, or would you prefer I come back later?"

**Offering choices and respecting autonomy** includes seemingly small decisions that convey respect: "Would you like to talk here or in a more private space?" "Would it help to have family present for this conversation?" "I have some questions about your living situation. Are you comfortable talking about that now?"

**Validating emotional responses** normalizes reactions and reduces shame: "Many people feel angry when they lose control over their body."

"It makes sense to feel scared given what you've been through."

"Your reactions are normal responses to abnormal events."

**Pacing and checking in** involves monitoring patient distress and adjusting your approach accordingly. Notice body language, affect changes, or withdrawal. Ask, "How are you doing with this conversation? Do you need a break?" Slow down when needed.

**Avoiding triggering language or scenarios** means being thoughtful about words and situations that might activate trauma. For abuse survivors, avoid using language such as "You have to..." or positioning yourself between the patient and the door. Acknowledge that for those with medical trauma, procedures may feel scary.

**Transparency about limitations and mandated reporting** at the outset builds trust better than surprising patients later. Explain confidentiality limits: "Most of what we discuss is confidential, but I'm required to report if I become concerned about abuse or neglect or if someone is in immediate danger."

**Collaborative safety planning** when patients express suicidal thoughts or concerning behaviors involves asking "What's helped you stay safe in the past?" and "What can we put in place to help you now?" rather than immediately resorting to involuntary interventions. Coercive responses should be last resorts, not first responses.

## Addressing Organizational Trauma and System-Level Practice

Individual trauma-informed practice, while essential, achieves limited impact within organizational systems that function in traumatizing ways. Trauma-informed care ideally extends to organizational policies, physical environments, and staff support systems (Bloom & Farragher, 2013).

**Organizational trauma-informed practice includes**

- physical environments that feel safe, not institutional or prisonlike
- policies that maximize patient choice and minimize coercion
- staff training in trauma-informed approaches
- attention to diversity, equity, and inclusion reducing identity-based trauma
- support for staff experiencing vicarious trauma
- reduction of restraint and seclusion use
- family involvement as default rather than exception

Social workers can advocate for organizational trauma-informed change through ethics committees, policy development participation, staff education, and documentation of how current practices cause harm.

## Vicarious Trauma and Secondary Traumatic Stress

Working with traumatized populations exposes social workers to vicarious trauma (trauma symptoms developing from hearing patients' trauma narratives) and secondary traumatic stress (stress reactions mirroring PTSD; Figley, 1995). These occupational hazards require recognition and active management.

**Signs of vicarious trauma include**

- intrusive thoughts about patients' trauma
- emotional numbing or detachment
- hypervigilance or exaggerated startle response
- cynicism or hopelessness about the world
- difficulty maintaining boundaries
- sleep disturbance
- physical symptoms (headaches, gastrointestinal problems)

**Protective strategies include**

- regular clinical supervision addressing emotional impacts
- peer support and debriefing
- maintaining boundaries between work and personal life
- self-care practices addressing physical, emotional, and spiritual needs
- limiting exposure through caseload diversity when possible
- organizational support and trauma-informed supervision

Vicarious trauma represents an occupational risk, not a personal failing. Seeking support demonstrates professional competence, not weakness.

# Critical Thinking Questions

1. Analyze trauma-informed care as a paradigm shift in health care delivery. How does this framework challenge traditional biomedical models and professional authority structures? What organizational barriers typically impede trauma-informed transformation, and what change theories might guide implementation?
2. Examine the concept of "universal trauma precautions" from an ethical perspective. Does assuming potential trauma history in all patients represent appropriate clinical caution or problematic overgeneralization? How might this approach affect therapeutic relationships differently across diverse populations?
3. Critically evaluate the relationship between individual trauma-informed practice and systemic change. Can practitioners working within traumatizing systems truly provide trauma-informed care, or does authentic trauma-informed practice require organizational transformation? Support your position with relevant literature.
4. Consider vicarious trauma and secondary traumatic stress through the lens of occupational health and professional ethics. What institutional responsibilities do health care organizations bear for supporting practitioners exposed to trauma, and how do current support systems reflect or contradict stated commitments to trauma-informed care?

# Key Takeaways

- Trauma profoundly affects physical and mental health, with traumatic experiences being common across patient populations.
- Health care settings can inadvertently re-traumatize patients through power dynamics, loss of control, and dismissive treatment.
- Six trauma-informed principles (safety, trustworthiness, peer support, collaboration, empowerment, cultural responsiveness) guide practice transformation.
- Trauma responses including hyperarousal, dissociation, avoidance, and control-seeking may be misinterpreted as personality pathology or noncompliance.
- Trauma-informed communication emphasizes transparency, choice, validation, pacing, and collaborative approaches.
- Vicarious trauma and secondary traumatic stress affect practitioners working with traumatized populations, requiring intentional self-care and support.

# Section I References


Agency for Healthcare Research and Quality. (2015). *Health literacy universal precautions toolkit* (2nd ed.). AHRQ Publication No. 15-0023-EF.

Alzheimer's Association. (2023). 2023 Alzheimer's disease facts and figures. *Alzheimer's & Dementia, 19*(4), 1598–1695. https://doi.org/10.1002/alz.13016

American Diabetes Association. (2023). Standards of medical care in diabetes—2023. *Diabetes Care, 46*(Supplement 1), S1–S4. https://doi.org/10.2337/dc23-Sint

Berkman, N. D., Sheridan, S. L., Donahue, K. E., Halpern, D. J., & Crotty, K. (2011). Low health literacy and health outcomes: An updated systematic review. *Annals of Internal Medicine, 155*(2), 97–107. https://doi.org/10.7326/0003-4819-155-2-201107190-00005

Berkowitz, S. A., Seligman, H. K., & Choudhry, N. K. (2014). Treat or eat: Food insecurity, cost-related medication underuse, and unmet needs. *American Journal of Medicine, 127*(4), 303–310. https://doi.org/10.1016/j.amjmed.2014.01.002

Bogo, M. (2015). *Field education for professional expertise: Integrating field and classroom learning*. Columbia University Press.

Borrell-Carrió, F., Suchman, A. L., & Epstein, R. M. (2004). The biopsychosocial model 25 years later: Principles, practice, and scientific inquiry. *Annals of Family Medicine, 2*(6), 576–582. https://doi.org/10.1370/afm.245

Bronstein, L. R. (2003). A model for interdisciplinary collaboration. *Social Work, 48*(3), 297–306. https://doi.org/10.1093/sw/48.3.297

Burau, V., & Blank, R. H. (2006). Comparing health policy: An assessment of typologies of health systems. *Journal of Comparative Policy Analysis, 8*(1), 63–76. https://doi.org/10.1080/13876980500513558

Bywaters, P., & McLeod, E. (1996). *Working for equality in health*. Routledge.

Cohen, S. (2004). Social relationships and health. *American Psychologist, 59*(8), 676–684. https://doi.org/10.1037/0003-066X.59.8.676

Coleman, E. A., Parry, C., Chalmers, S., & Min, S. J. (2006). The care transitions intervention: Results of a randomized controlled trial. *Archives of Internal Medicine, 166*(17), 1822–1828. https://doi.org/10.1001/archinte.166.17.1822

D'Amour, D., Ferrada-Videla, M., San Martin Rodriguez, L., & Beaulieu, M. D. (2005). The conceptual basis for interprofessional collaboration: Core concepts and theoretical frameworks. *Journal of Interprofessional Care, 19*(Supplement 1), 116–131. https://doi.org/10.1080/13561820500082529

Dziegielewski, S. F. (2013). *The changing face of health care social work: Opportunities and challenges for professional practice* (3rd ed.). Springer Publishing Company.

Engel, G. L. (1977). The need for a new medical model: A challenge for biomedicine. *Science, 196*(4286), 129–136. https://doi.org/10.1126/science.847460

Ewing, J. A. (1984). Detecting alcoholism: The CAGE questionnaire. *JAMA, 252*(14), 1905–1907. https://doi.org/10.1001/jama.1984.03350140051025

Figley, C. R. (Ed.). (1995). *Compassion fatigue: Coping with secondary traumatic stress disorder in those who treat the traumatized*. Brunner/Mazel.

Folstein, M. F., Folstein, S. E., & McHugh, P. R. (1975). "Mini-mental state": A practical method for grading the cognitive state of patients for the clinician. *Journal of Psychiatric Research, 12*(3), 189–198. https://doi.org/10.1016/0022-3956(75)90026-6

Global Initiative for Chronic Obstructive Lung Disease. (2023). *Global strategy for the diagnosis, management, and prevention of chronic obstructive pulmonary disease (2023 report)*. https://goldcopd.org

Granger, C. V., Hamilton, B. B., Linacre, J. M., Heinemann, A. W., & Wright, B. D. (1993). Performance profiles of the functional independence measure. *American Journal of Physical Medicine & Rehabilitation, 72*(2), 84–89. https://doi.org/10.1097/00002060-199304000-00005

Hepworth, D. H., Rooney, R. H., Rooney, G. D., & Strom-Gottfried, K. (2016). *Direct social work practice: Theory and skills* (10th ed.). Cengage Learning.

Hunt, S. A., Abraham, W. T., Chin, M. H., Feldman, A. M., Francis, G. S., Ganiats, T. G., Jessup, M., Konstam, M. A., Mancini, D. M., Michl, K., Oates, J. A., Rahko, P. S., Silver, M. A., Stevenson, L. W., Yancy, C. W., Antman, E. M., Smith, S. C., Jr., Adams, C. D., Anderson, J. L., Riegel, B. (2009). 2009 focused update incorporated into the ACC/AHA 2005 guidelines for the diagnosis and management of heart failure in adults. *Circulation, 119*(14), e391–e479. https://doi.org/10.1161/CIRCULATIONAHA.109.192065

Inouye, S. K., van Dyck, C. H., Alessi, C. A., Balkin, S., Siegal, A. P., & Horwitz, R. I. (1990). Clarifying confusion: The confusion assessment method. *Annals of Internal Medicine, 113*(12), 941–948. https://doi.org/10.7326/0003-4819-113-12-941

Institute of Medicine. (2011). *Relieving pain in America: A blueprint for transforming prevention, care, education, and research.* National Academies Press.

Jordan, C., & Franklin, C. (2011). *Clinical assessment for social workers: Quantitative and qualitative methods* (3rd ed.). Oxford University Press.

Katon, W. J. (2011). Epidemiology and treatment of depression in patients with chronic medical illness. *Dialogues in Clinical Neuroscience, 13*(1), 7–23. https://doi.org/10.31887/DCNS.2011.13.1/wkaton

Kramer, B. J., Kavanaugh, M., Trentham-Dietz, A., Walsh, M., & Yonker, J. A. (2013). Complicated grief symptoms in caregivers of persons with lung cancer: The role of family conflict, intrapsychic strains, and hospice utilization. *Omega, 62*(3), 201–220.

Section II

# The Heart of Patient and Family Care

The technical competencies explored in Section I provide essential foundations for medical social work practice. However, technical skill alone proves insufficient for effective practice. The heart of social work lies in the therapeutic relationship, the capacity to be fully present with individuals and families during vulnerable moments, and the commitment to honoring human dignity amid suffering and uncertainty.

This section examines the relational and supportive dimensions of medical social work practice, guided by patient-centered care principles that position the patient and family at the center of all clinical decisions (Institute of Medicine, 2001). Patient-centered care emphasizes respect for patient preferences, values, and needs; coordination and integration of care; clear information and communication; physical comfort and emotional support; involvement of family and friends; and continuity and transition management. These principles align closely with social work's person-in-environment perspective and strengths-based approaches.

Research consistently demonstrates that patient-centered care improves outcomes including increased patient satisfaction, better adherence to treatment plans, reduced anxiety and depression, improved functional status, and decreased health care utilization (Rathert et al., 2013). Social workers contribute uniquely to patient-centered care through psychosocial expertise, attention to family systems, cultural responsiveness, and advocacy for patient voices in treatment planning.

The five chapters that follow address core competencies in supportive care.

**Chapter 6: Crisis Intervention in Medical Settings** applies crisis theory to health care contexts, examining how social workers provide stabilization, support, and resource mobilization during acute crises including medical emergencies, traumatic diagnoses, and family conflicts.

**Chapter 7: Grief, Loss, and End-of-Life Support** explores contemporary grief theories and evidence-based approaches to supporting patients and families facing death and bereavement, including anticipatory grief, complicated grief, and cultural variations in mourning.

**Chapter 8: Practicing Cultural Competence in Health Care** examines cultural humility as an alternative to competence-based frameworks, addressing how social workers provide culturally responsive care that honors diverse health beliefs, communication patterns, and family structures.

**Chapter 9: Mastering Discharge Planning** presents evidence-based strategies for comprehensive discharge planning that addresses medical needs, functional limitations, social support, and social determinants of health to enable safe transitions and prevent readmissions.

**Chapter 10: Educating About Advance Directives** discusses the legal, ethical, and communication dimensions of advance care planning, exploring how social workers facilitate conversations about end-of-life preferences and decision-making.

These chapters emphasize that while medical treatment addresses disease, social work addresses the human experience of illness within complex social contexts. The capacity to sit with suffering, witness pain without fixing, and honor patient autonomy even during crisis represents the essence of social work's contribution to health care.

CHAPTER 6

# Crisis Intervention in Medical Settings

## Learning Objectives

By the end of this chapter, you will be able to do the following:

- Apply crisis intervention theoretical frameworks to medical settings
- Assess crisis severity and intervention needs systematically
- Implement evidence-based crisis stabilization strategies
- Distinguish between crisis intervention and ongoing psychotherapy
- Maintain professional boundaries and emotional regulation during high-intensity encounters

## Understanding Crisis in Health Care Contexts

Crisis represents a state of psychological disequilibrium occurring when individuals confront situations that exceed their usual coping capacities, creating temporary inability to function effectively (Caplan, 1964; Roberts, 2005). Crises emerge not solely from events themselves but from the interaction between events, available resources, and perception of threat. An event constituting crisis for one individual may represent a manageable stressor for another, depending on factors including previous trauma exposure, social support, coping skills, cultural meaning-making, and concurrent stressors (James & Gilliland, 2017).

Health care settings generate numerous crisis-inducing situations: sudden life-threatening diagnoses, unexpected surgical complications, traumatic injuries, death of a loved one, and overwhelming treatment demands. Medical crises differ from other crisis types in several ways. First, they occur within institutional environments characterized by unfamiliarity, loss of privacy, and reduced control. Second, they often involve physical pain or impairment that complicates emotional processing. Third, they require rapid decision-making about treatment options with insufficient time for deliberation. Fourth, they typically impact entire family systems rather than individuals alone (Kleespies, 2009).

Crisis intervention in medical settings serves several functions: emotional stabilization, practical problem-solving, resource mobilization, and restoration of equilibrium sufficient for adaptive functioning. Unlike ongoing psychotherapy focused on personality change or deep insight, crisis intervention emphasizes here-and-now support, concrete assistance, and time-limited engagement (Roberts, 2005). The goal involves returning individuals to pre-crisis functioning levels or, ideally, slightly improved functioning through development of new coping strategies.

Research supports crisis intervention effectiveness across diverse populations and settings. Systematic reviews demonstrate that brief crisis interventions reduce psychological distress, prevent psychiatric hospitalizations, and improve problem-solving capacity (Roberts & Everly, 2006). In medical settings specifically, social work crisis intervention contributes to improved patient satisfaction, reduced lengths of stay, and enhanced family coping (Beder, 2006).

## Theoretical Frameworks for Crisis Intervention

Multiple theoretical perspectives inform crisis intervention practice, each offering particular insights into crisis dynamics and intervention strategies.

**Crisis theory** (Caplan, 1964) conceptualizes crisis as a temporary state of upset and disorganization characterized by inability to use usual problem-solving methods. Caplan identified four phases of crisis development: initial rise in tension from precipitating event, failure of usual coping methods, further tension rise prompting emergency problem-solving efforts, and either crisis resolution or serious personality disorganization if no solution emerges. This framework emphasizes that crisis presents both danger and opportunity. While crises create vulnerability to psychological harm, they also create openness to change and potential for growth through development of new coping strategies.

**Roberts's seven-stage crisis intervention model** (2005) provides a structured approach particularly applicable to medical settings:

1. Plan and conduct thorough biopsychosocial and lethality assessment
2. Establish rapport and rapidly establish collaborative relationship
3. Identify major problems including precipitating events
4. Encourage exploration of feelings and emotions
5. Generate and explore alternatives and untapped coping resources
6. Restore functioning through action plan implementation
7. Follow up to evaluate outcomes and referrals

This model emphasizes systematic assessment while maintaining flexibility to address presenting needs. The seven stages may occur sequentially or recursively depending on crisis dynamics and patient responses.

**ABC model of crisis intervention** (Kanel, 2019) simplifies crisis response into three components: A (achieving rapport), B (boiling down the problem to basics), and C (coping strategies). This streamlined approach proves particularly useful in fast-paced medical environments where comprehensive assessment may be impossible. The ABC model prioritizes rapid relationship building, problem clarification, and identification of immediate coping strategies.

**Psychological First Aid** (Brymer et al., 2006), developed for disaster response but applicable to medical crises, emphasizes eight core actions: contact and engagement, safety and comfort, stabilization, information gathering, practical assistance, connection with social supports, information on coping, and linkage with collaborative services. This framework explicitly avoids pathologizing normal crisis reactions and focuses on supportive presence rather than clinical intervention.

## The ABCDE Crisis Assessment Framework

Systematic assessment provides the foundation for effective crisis intervention. The ABCDE framework offers a memorable structure for comprehensive yet efficient crisis assessment in medical settings (Kleespies, 2009):

**A: Assess for danger** evaluates immediate safety risks including suicidal ideation, homicidal thoughts, psychotic symptoms, severe substance intoxication or withdrawal, and risk of elopement from medical care. Lethality assessment requires direct questioning: "Are you having thoughts of hurting yourself or ending your life?" "Do you have a plan?" "What has kept you from acting on these thoughts?"

Positive responses necessitate immediate safety interventions including constant observation, psychiatric consultation, and voluntary or involuntary psychiatric hold when indicated.

Safety assessment extends beyond self-harm to include abuse, neglect, and domestic violence. Questions such as "Do you feel safe at home?" and "Has anyone hurt you or threatened you?" screen for interpersonal violence requiring mandated reporting and safety planning.

**B: Build rapport and establish therapeutic alliance** recognizes that crisis intervention effectiveness depends on rapid relationship development. Strategies include introducing yourself clearly and explaining your role, expressing empathy and normalizing distress, offering privacy and comfortable space when possible, using active listening with minimal interruption, respecting cultural norms regarding eye contact and personal space, and asking permission to discuss sensitive topics.

Rapport building in crisis differs from traditional therapeutic relationship development due to time constraints and urgency. Social workers must convey genuine care and trustworthiness quickly, often within minutes rather than sessions.

**C: Contain emotions and provide support** involves creating space for emotional expression while preventing overwhelming dysregulation. Techniques include validation of feelings without judgment, normalization of crisis reactions, grounding exercises for severe anxiety or dissociation, psychoeducation about stress responses, and encouragement of healthy emotional expression.

Emotional containment does not mean suppressing feelings but rather helping individuals experience emotions without being overwhelmed. This balance proves particularly challenging in medical crises where raw grief, terror, and anger naturally emerge.

**D: Develop problem-solving plan** shifts from emotional processing to practical action. Crisis intervention emphasizes concrete, immediate steps rather than comprehensive long-term planning. Questions that facilitate problem-solving include: "What is your most pressing concern right now?" "What has helped in difficult situations before?" "Who can you reach out to for support?" "What feels manageable to address today?"

Problem-solving during crisis prioritizes achievable goals that restore sense of control. Rather than tackling every identified problem, focus on one or two immediate concerns amenable to action.

**E: Engage resources and follow-up** connects individuals with supports including family and friends, community resources, mental health services, spiritual care, peer support groups, and medical team members. Resource engagement during crisis prevents isolation and mobilizes ongoing support after social work contact ends.

Follow-up, when feasible, demonstrates continued care and evaluates intervention effectiveness. Even brief check-ins communicate that the person matters and strengthens therapeutic relationships.

## Common Crisis Scenarios in Medical Settings

Medical social workers encounter diverse crisis presentations requiring flexible application of intervention principles. Understanding common scenarios enables anticipatory planning and efficient response.

**Sudden terminal diagnosis** confronts patients and families with mortality in unexpected ways. A person who arrived at the emergency department with vague symptoms learns they have advanced, untreatable cancer. Crisis intervention addresses

- acute grief and shock reactions
- information needs regarding prognosis and options
- family notification and support
- advance care planning initiation
- connection with palliative care services
- processing existential and spiritual concerns

**Traumatic injury or sudden disability** creates immediate functional loss and identity disruption. The young adult paralyzed in a car accident or the active elder who suffers disabling stroke faces radical life changes. Intervention focuses on:

- acute adjustment support
- grief over lost abilities
- family system impact and caregiver support
- rehabilitation planning and goal-setting
- peer support and disability community connection
- addressing hopelessness and suicidal ideation

**Neonatal loss or complicated birth** devastates parents' hopes and expectations. The stillbirth, severe birth injury, or NICU admission triggers complex grief. Social work response includes:

- anticipatory grief support
- memory-making and ritual facilitation
- couples counseling regarding different grieving styles
- sibling support if other children present
- connection with perinatal loss support groups
- follow-up bereavement services

**Family conflict regarding treatment decisions** occurs when family members disagree about aggressive treatment versus comfort care, often complicated by family dynamics predating the medical crisis. Intervention strategies include

- individual meetings with key family members
- facilitated family conferences
- clarification of patient's previously expressed wishes
- mediation when family relationships allow
- ethics consultation when conflicts persist
- legal clarification of surrogate authority

**Domestic violence disclosure during hospitalization** creates safety crises requiring immediate response. When patients disclose abuse while admitted, social workers must

- ensure immediate safety within hospital
- complete mandatory abuse reporting
- provide safety planning before discharge
- connect with domestic violence advocates
- address perpetrator access and visitation
- coordinate with law enforcement when indicated

**Psychiatric emergency in medical patient** involves suicide attempts during medical admission, severe anxiety or panic, psychotic symptoms, or behavioral dysregulation. Response includes:

- immediate safety assessment and monitoring
- psychiatric consultation
- medication evaluation
- family psychoeducation
- voluntary or involuntary psychiatric hold processing
- transition planning to psychiatric care

## Self-Regulation and Professional Boundaries

Crisis intervention work generates intense emotional responses in practitioners. Witnessing suffering, absorbing others' distress, and functioning amid chaos creates risks of vicarious trauma, compassion fatigue, and boundary violations (Figley, 1995). Effective crisis intervention requires attending to your own regulation while supporting others.

**Grounding and centering techniques** help social workers maintain presence during emotional encounters. Strategies include focused breathing, physical grounding through feet contact with floor, brief muscle tension and release, and internal calming self-statements. Practice these techniques outside crisis situations so they become automatic during high-stress encounters.

**Emotional awareness and management** involve noticing your reactions without being controlled by them. When feeling overwhelmed, anxious, or angry, brief self-inquiry helps: "What am I feeling?"

"What triggered this reaction?"

"What do I need right now?"

Sometimes simply naming the emotion reduces its intensity.

**Professional boundaries in crisis** require particular attention because crises evoke helping instincts that may exceed professional role limits. Appropriate boundaries include

- limiting contact to professional context and work hours
- avoiding personal relationship development with patients
- referring needs outside your scope to appropriate resources
- recognizing when your own trauma responses interfere with objectivity
- seeking consultation when emotionally activated

Boundaries do not mean coldness or detachment but rather maintaining clarity about your role, limits, and therapeutic relationship parameters.

**Debriefing and Support** after intense crisis interventions prevents cumulative trauma. Options include peer consultation, clinical supervision, structured debriefing protocols after critical incidents, and personal therapy when indicated. Organizations should provide debriefing opportunities after particularly traumatic events such as patient deaths, violence, or mass casualties.

## Distinguishing Crisis Intervention from Ongoing Therapy

Crisis intervention represents a distinct practice modality rather than abbreviated therapy. Understanding these differences prevents scope creep and clarifies referral needs (Roberts, 2005):

| Crisis Intervention | Psychotherapy |
|---|---|
| Time-limited (1–6 contacts) | Ongoing (weeks to years) |
| Present-focused | Past and present focused |
| Problem-solving emphasis | Insight and personality change |
| Active, directive approach | More reflective, client-directed |
| Practical assistance | Primarily verbal processing |
| Any appropriate setting | Designated therapeutic space |
| Restoration of baseline function | Growth beyond baseline |

When patients require ongoing mental health support beyond crisis stabilization, appropriate referrals to outpatient therapy, psychiatry, or community mental health services become essential. Crisis intervention establishes immediate safety and functioning; ongoing therapy addresses underlying vulnerabilities and promotes lasting change.

## Critical Thinking Questions

1. Analyze crisis intervention from a critical theory perspective. How might traditional crisis models reflect particular cultural assumptions about emotional expression, family involvement, and appropriate help-seeking? What modifications would make crisis intervention more culturally responsive across diverse populations?
2. Evaluate the tension between rapid crisis assessment necessitated by health care time constraints and thorough psychosocial evaluation required for safe intervention. How do institutional pressures for efficiency potentially compromise crisis intervention quality, and what advocacy strategies might address these structural barriers?
3. Examine the concept of "crisis" as socially constructed rather than objectively defined. How do factors including race, class, gender, and disability status influence which situations health care systems recognize as crises versus expected stressors? What implications does this have for equitable crisis service provision?
4. Critically assess the evidence base for crisis intervention effectiveness. What methodological challenges complicate research on crisis intervention outcomes, and how might these limitations affect confidence in recommended practices? What gaps in crisis intervention research most urgently require attention?

## Key Takeaways

- Crisis represents psychological disequilibrium when situations exceed usual coping capacities, creating both vulnerability and opportunity for growth.

- Multiple theoretical frameworks (Roberts's seven-stage model, ABC model, psychological first aid) inform crisis intervention, emphasizing systematic assessment, rapport building, and time-limited support.
- The ABCDE framework provides comprehensive yet efficient crisis assessment structure addressing danger, rapport, emotional containment, problem-solving, and resource engagement.
- Common medical crises include terminal diagnoses, traumatic injuries, neonatal loss, family conflicts, domestic violence disclosure, and psychiatric emergencies.
- Practitioner self-regulation, emotional awareness, and clear professional boundaries prove essential for sustainable crisis intervention practice.
- Crisis intervention differs fundamentally from psychotherapy in time frame, focus, goals, and intervention strategies.

CHAPTER 7

# Grief, Loss, and End-of-Life Support

## Learning Objectives

By the end of this chapter, you will be able to do the following:

- Apply contemporary grief theories to understand diverse mourning responses
- Distinguish between normative grief and complicated grief requiring specialized intervention
- Provide evidence-based support for anticipatory grief in progressive illness
- Navigate cultural and spiritual dimensions of dying and bereavement
- Implement self-care strategies when repeatedly exposed to death and loss

## Contemporary Understanding of Grief and Bereavement

Grief, the natural response to loss, encompasses physical, emotional, cognitive, behavioral, social, and spiritual dimensions (Stroebe & Schut, 2010). While often discussed in relation to death, grief occurs in response to numerous losses including disability, independence, relationships, roles, and hopes for the future. Medical social workers encounter grief in all its forms, requiring theoretical understanding and practice skills that honor diverse grief expressions while identifying concerning patterns requiring intervention.

Historical grief theories emphasized stage or phase models, most notably Kübler-Ross's (1969) five stages of dying: denial, anger, bargaining, depression, acceptance. While these frameworks generated important awareness of dying experiences, contemporary research reveals that grief does not follow predictable linear progression. Individuals move fluidly between different emotional states, experience multiple reactions simultaneously, and display highly individualized mourning patterns influenced by factors including relationship to the deceased, circumstances of death, cultural background, spiritual beliefs, previous loss experiences, and concurrent stressors (Neimeyer, 2001).

Current grief theories conceptualize mourning as active meaning-making process rather than passive emotional experience requiring "completion." This paradigm shift has profound practice implications, moving social workers from encouraging "closure" or "moving on" toward supporting continuing bonds, narrative reconstruction, and meaning-making that integrates loss into ongoing life (Klass et al., 1996).

Research distinguishes between acute grief, the intense early mourning period typically lasting months; integrated grief, the adaptation that allows resuming life while maintaining connection to the deceased; and prolonged or complicated grief, which is a persistent, intense grief that significantly impairs functioning beyond typical timeframes (Shear, 2015). Approximately 7%–10% of bereaved individuals develop complicated grief requiring specialized treatment (Prigerson et al., 2009).

## The Dual Process Model of Coping With Bereavement

The dual process model (Stroebe & Schut, 1999, 2010) provides a nuanced framework for understanding grief that guides social work support. This model proposes that bereaved individuals oscillate between two types of coping:

**Loss-oriented coping** involves confronting the loss directly through activities such as crying, yearning, looking at photographs, talking about the deceased, and experiencing grief waves. This emotional processing proves necessary for integrating loss.

**Restoration-oriented coping** focuses on managing life changes resulting from loss, including assuming new roles, developing new routines, distracting from grief, and attending to practical demands. This forward-looking orientation enables continuing life.

Healthy grief involves movement between both orientations rather than exclusive focus on either. Cultural and individual factors influence the balance between loss and restoration focus. Some mourners spend more time in loss orientation, while others prefer restoration activities. Neither approach proves universally superior; rather, flexibility to engage both types of coping and oscillation between them predicts adaptive outcomes (Stroebe & Schut, 2010).

The dual process model has important practice implications. Social workers should not interpret restoration-oriented behavior (returning to work quickly, avoiding grief conversations, keeping busy) as denial or avoidance requiring correction. Similarly, intense emotional expression should not be labeled as "dwelling" or "stuck." Instead, social workers support clients' current coping approach while gently encouraging oscillation if someone remains exclusively in one orientation.

## Worden's Tasks of Mourning

William Worden's (2018) task-based model conceptualizes mourning as active process rather than passive experience, emphasizing bereaved individuals' agency. There are four tasks.

**Task I: Accept the reality of the loss** involves coming to terms intellectually and emotionally that the person has died and will not return. This acceptance does not occur instantly but gradually through repeated confrontations with the reality of absence.

**Task II: Process the pain of grief** acknowledges that avoiding or suppressing grief creates long-term complications. While the specific pain experienced varies, working through emotional responses proves necessary. However, the timing and manner of processing differ individually and culturally.

**Task III: Adjust to a world without the deceased** encompasses multiple adjustments including external (practical life changes), internal (sense of self), and spiritual (belief systems and meaning). Widows learn to manage previously shared responsibilities; parents losing children grapple with shattered worldviews; and adults losing parents reassess mortality and family roles.

**Task IV: Find an enduring connection while embarking on new life** modifies earlier conceptualizations encouraging "letting go." Contemporary understanding recognizes that maintaining ongoing connection to deceased loved ones through memory, legacy, values, and spiritual beliefs proves healthy. The task involves finding appropriate place for the deceased in emotional life while moving forward with living.

Worden emphasizes that these tasks occur non-linearly, require varying timeframes, and may be revisited throughout life at significant moments (anniversaries, holidays, milestones). Social workers guide task engagement without imposing timelines or prescriptive approaches.

## Anticipatory Grief in Progressive Illness

Anticipatory grief occurs before death when loss appears inevitable, common in progressive illnesses such as dementia, cancer, and heart failure (Rando, 2000). This grief encompasses mourning for multiple losses: impending death, declining function, changing relationship dynamics, and surrendered hopes for the future.

Research reveals that anticipatory grief differs qualitatively from post-death grief. While some aspects prove similar, the ambiguity of ongoing deterioration without definitive endpoint creates unique challenges. Caregivers and patients may experience relief alternating with guilt, exhaustion alongside devotion, and detachment mixed with desperate clinging (Holley & Mast, 2009).

Important findings about anticipatory grief include the following:

1. **Anticipatory grief does not reduce post-death grief:** Early theories proposed that mourning before death would diminish bereavement intensity. Research refutes this, demonstrating that pre-death grief does not immunize against post-death mourning. However, anticipatory grief may facilitate certain practical preparations and relationship resolutions (Rando, 2000).
2. **Premature detachment risks exist:** Caregivers experiencing prolonged anticipatory grief may emotionally withdraw before death occurs, creating guilt and complicated bereavement. Social workers help caregivers maintain connection while acknowledging losses already experienced.
3. **Disenfranchised anticipatory grief** affects caregivers whose grief receives limited social recognition because the person "hasn't died yet." Support systems may expect cheerfulness and hope, invalidating grief responses to ongoing deterioration (Doka, 2002).
4. **Ambiguous loss** characterizes dementia particularly, where the person's physical presence continues while personality, recognition, and relationship qualities disappear. This creates profound confusion and prevents grief resolution typical when death provides finality (Boss, 2011).

Social work interventions for anticipatory grief include

- normalizing and validating grief responses to ongoing losses
- facilitating legacy activities (memory boxes, letters, life review)
- supporting relationship maintenance despite changes
- addressing caregiver guilt about emotions including relief or wishing for death
- respite care to prevent caregiver exhaustion
- advance care planning conversations
- connection with support groups for specific conditions
- preparation for death while maintaining hope for quality time

## Complicated Grief: Recognition and Response

Most bereaved individuals adapt to loss without professional mental health intervention, supported by natural social networks and spiritual communities. However, a subset develops complicated grief (also termed prolonged grief disorder or persistent complex bereavement disorder), characterized by intense yearning, preoccupation with the deceased, difficulty accepting death, bitterness, numbness, meaninglessness, and severe functional impairment persisting beyond normative timeframes (Prigerson et al., 2009; Shear, 2015).

**Risk factors for complicated grief** include

- sudden, unexpected, or traumatic death
- death of a child or young person
- highly dependent or ambivalent relationship with deceased

- previous psychiatric history, especially depression or anxiety
- multiple concurrent losses
- lack of social support
- secondary losses (financial hardship, housing instability)
- inability to engage in mourning rituals

**Screening for complicated grief** uses validated instruments including the Prolonged Grief Disorder scale (PG-13) and the Inventory of Complicated Grief (ICG). Key screening questions include the following:

"Do you feel stuck in your grief?"

"Are you having persistent, intrusive thoughts about your loss?"

"Has grief prevented you from resuming daily activities and relationships?"

**Specialized Treatment** for complicated grief differs from traditional grief counseling or general psychotherapy. Complicated grief treatment (CGT), an evidence-based manualized intervention, combines elements of cognitive-behavioral therapy and interpersonal therapy specifically targeting complicated grief symptoms (Shear et al., 2016). CGT includes

- revisiting the death story to reduce avoidance
- imaginal conversations with the deceased
- goals for re-engagement with life
- memory work distinguishing healthy remembering from painful yearning

Social workers identifying complicated grief should refer to mental health specialists trained in CGT while providing supportive counseling and care coordination.

## Cultural and Spiritual Dimensions of Death and Dying

Culture profoundly influences grief expressions, mourning rituals, beliefs about death and afterlife, family involvement in dying processes, and appropriate practitioner roles (Rosenblatt, 2008). Social workers must approach cultural differences with humility, avoiding assumptions while seeking to understand each family's unique traditions and needs.

**Common cultural variations** include

1. **Emotional expression norms:** Some cultures value open grief displays including wailing, while others prize emotional restraint and private mourning. Neither approach proves more "healthy" both represent culturally appropriate grief.
2. **Family decision-making:** Individualistic Western cultures typically emphasize patient autonomy in end-of-life decisions. Collectivist cultures may prioritize family consensus, with some families preferring to protect dying individuals from prognostic information.
3. **Death location preferences:** While hospice ideology promotes home death, some cultures view hospital death as showing appropriate use of all available resources. Others strongly prefer home to enable proper rituals.
4. **Body handling and funeral practices:** Diverse traditions govern body preparation, viewing practices, burial timing, cremation acceptability, and mourning period lengths. Religious and cultural leaders provide guidance on acceptable practices.
5. **Afterlife beliefs:** Concepts of heaven, reincarnation, ancestral spirits, or nonexistence shape how individuals approach death and find meaning in loss.
6. **Communication about death:** Some languages and cultures avoid direct death language, preferring euphemisms or indirect communication. Western medicine's preference for explicit prognostic disclosure conflicts with cultures valuing indirection and hope maintenance.

**Culturally responsive practice** requires asking rather than assuming:

"Are there cultural or religious practices important to you during this time?"

"How does your family usually make medical decisions?"

"What rituals or traditions would you like us to support?"

Partner with chaplains, cultural liaisons, or community religious leaders to understand and accommodate varied practices.

## Social Work Roles at End of Life

Palliative social workers provide specialized services to patients with serious illness and their families, addressing psychosocial dimensions of dying, bereavement, and care coordination (National Association of Social Workers, 2004). Core competencies include (Kramer et al., 2013)

**Advance care planning facilitation** involves conversations about values, preferences, and goals of care to guide future medical decisions. Social workers help patients articulate what quality of life means, identify acceptable trade-offs between longevity and comfort, designate surrogate decision-makers, and complete advance directive documentation. These conversations require skill in addressing emotions that arise when contemplating mortality while ensuring understanding of medical options.

**Family conferences** convene interdisciplinary teams and families to discuss prognosis, treatment options, and goals of care. Social workers often facilitate these difficult conversations, managing family dynamics, translating medical information, attending to emotional responses, and ensuring all voices are heard. Skilled facilitation prevents family conflicts and supports consensus building.

**Grief and bereavement counseling** provides emotional support through anticipatory grief, active dying, and bereavement. Interventions include validating grief responses, facilitating meaning-making, addressing guilt and regret, supporting continuing bonds, and providing grief education. Social workers assess for complicated grief and refer for specialized treatment when indicated.

**Practical support and resource coordination** addresses concrete needs, including hospice enrollment, financial assistance, respite care, funeral planning, and estate issues. Dying patients and families face overwhelming practical demands alongside emotional distress. Social work navigation reduces burden and ensures needs are met.

**Legacy and life review work** helps patients reflect on life meaning, relationships, and values. Activities include recording life stories, creating memory books, writing letters to loved ones, and identifying legacies. This meaning-making work provides comfort and leaves tangible remembrances for survivors (Keall et al., 2013).

**Ethical consultation** occurs when conflicts arise regarding treatment decisions, usually between aggressive intervention and comfort care. Social workers participate in ethics committees, advocate for patient preferences, mediate family disagreements, and ensure vulnerable patients' voices are heard.

**Staff support** recognizes that repeated exposure to death affects healthcare professionals. Social workers provide debriefing, facilitate staff memorials, and educate about vicarious trauma and self-care.

## Practitioner Self-Care in Death Work

Regular exposure to death and grieving families creates occupational hazards including compassion fatigue, vicarious traumatization, existential distress, and anticipatory anxiety about one's own mortality and losses (Papadatou, 2009). Sustainable practice requires intentional self-care and organizational support.

**Normalize emotional responses** to death work rather than interpreting distress as professional weakness. Sadness after patient deaths, anxiety when facing difficult family meetings, and emotional numbing during busy periods represent normal reactions to abnormal repeated loss exposure.

**Create transition rituals** between work and personal life. Physical or mental rituals that signal work ending help prevent carrying death preoccupation home. Examples include changing clothes, specific music, exercise, or visualization of leaving work concerns at the workplace.

**Maintain meaning and purpose** through regular reflection on why this work matters and how it serves values. Journaling, supervision conversations, or peer discussions that revisit professional purpose sustain commitment during difficult periods.

**Diversify caseload when possible** to prevent exclusive focus on dying patients. Some settings allow rotation between hospice and non-hospice patients, providing relief from constant death exposure.

**Engage personal grief work** through therapy, spiritual direction, or support groups. Unresolved personal losses may be activated by professional death encounters, requiring attention separate from workplace support.

**Build community and peer support** through case consultation groups, peer supervision, or informal colleague connections. Sharing difficult experiences with those who understand provides validation and perspective.

**Organizational responsibility** extends beyond individual self-care to structural support including reasonable caseloads, access to supervision, debriefing after traumatic deaths, training in self-care, and culture that values practitioner wellness alongside patient care.

## Critical Thinking Questions

1. Critique the concept of "closure" in grief discourse. How does this language reflect particular cultural values about emotional resolution and linear progression? What alternative frameworks better honor diverse and non-linear grief experiences?
2. Analyze anticipatory grief through the lens of ambiguous loss theory. How does this theoretical perspective enhance understanding of grief in dementia caregiving specifically, and what practice implications emerge from this analysis?
3. Examine the evidence base for complicated grief treatment. What assumptions about healthy grief underlie the designation of certain mourning patterns as "complicated" or "prolonged"? How might cultural factors influence diagnostic thresholds for pathological grief?
4. Evaluate the tension between patient-centered advance care planning emphasizing individual autonomy and family-centered decision-making valued in collectivist cultures. How can social workers navigate this conflict without imposing Western values while ensuring patient protection? What ethical frameworks guide resolution of these competing commitments?

## Key Takeaways

- Contemporary grief theory conceptualizes mourning as active meaning-making rather than passive emotional experience requiring completion.
- The dual process model and Worden's tasks of mourning provide frameworks that honor individualized grief while identifying concerning patterns.
- Anticipatory grief in progressive illness creates unique challenges including ambiguous loss, disenfranchisement, and caregiver exhaustion requiring specialized support.
- Complicated grief affects approximately 7%–10% of bereaved individuals, requiring recognition and referral to evidence-based specialized treatment.
- Cultural and spiritual dimensions of death profoundly shape dying experiences, mourning practices, and appropriate social work roles, requiring cultural humility and individualized approaches.

- Sustainable end-of-life practice requires intentional self-care strategies and organizational support addressing repeated death exposure impacts.

CHAPTER 8

# Practicing Cultural Competence in Healthcare

## Learning Objectives

By the end of this chapter, you will be able to do the following:

- Distinguish between cultural competence and cultural humility frameworks
- Analyze how culture shapes health beliefs, treatment preferences, and family dynamics
- Implement culturally responsive assessment and intervention strategies
- Navigate language access requirements and interpreter utilization
- Address implicit bias and structural racism in health care delivery

## From Cultural Competence to Cultural Humility

Health care literature historically emphasized cultural competence, defined as possessing knowledge, awareness, and skills to work effectively with diverse populations (Betancourt et al., 2003). This framework generated important attention to cultural factors in health and illness. However, critics argue that competence-based approaches risk several problems: suggesting mastery of entire cultures is achievable, essentializing and stereotyping cultural groups, positioning culture as static rather than dynamic, and maintaining power imbalances by positioning practitioners as experts (Tervalon & Murray-García, 1998; Hook et al., 2013).

**Cultural humility** emerged as an alternative paradigm emphasizing lifelong learning and critical self-reflection rather than competence achievement (Tervalon & Murray-García, 1998). This framework rests on three principles:

1. **Lifelong Learning and critical self-reflection** acknowledges that complete understanding of any culture other than one's own remains impossible. Practitioners must maintain openness to learning from each patient and family, recognizing individual variations within cultural groups. Critical self-reflection involves examining one's own cultural assumptions, biases, and privileges that shape clinical perceptions and interactions (Hook et al., 2013).
2. **Challenging power imbalances** requires recognizing that health care relationships inherently contain power differentials between providers and patients. Cultural humility actively works to minimize these imbalances through patient-centered care, shared decision-making, and honoring patient expertise about their own lives. This proves particularly critical when cultural differences intersect with existing power disparities based on race, class, language, immigration status, or other marginalized identities.
3. **Institutional accountability** extends cultural responsiveness beyond individual practitioner behav-

iors to organizational policies, procedures, and practices. Institutions demonstrate cultural humility through diverse workforce recruitment, language access services, culturally appropriate patient education materials, community partnerships, and systematic assessment of health disparities. Individual cultural humility proves insufficient without institutional commitment (Foronda et al., 2016).

Research supports cultural humility's benefits. Studies link cultural humility to improved patient satisfaction, better treatment adherence, reduced health disparities, and enhanced therapeutic relationships (Hook et al., 2013; Yeager & Bauer-Wu, 2013). Patients report feeling more respected and understood by culturally humble practitioners compared to those claiming cultural competence.

For social workers, cultural humility aligns closely with core professional values including respect for dignity and worth, importance of relationships, and commitment to social justice. The shift from competence to humility reframes cultural responsiveness as an ongoing ethical commitment rather than a skill set to master.

## Culture's Influence on Health and Health Care

Culture encompasses shared beliefs, values, customs, and behaviors transmitted across generations that shape worldview and identity (Kleinman & Benson, 2006). Some cultural influences on health care are as follows.

**Health belief systems** involve disease causation (biomedical, spiritual, energetic imbalance, punishment, karma), appropriate treatments (Western medicine, traditional healing, prayer, herbs), prevention practices, and body conceptualizations. These beliefs profoundly affect treatment acceptance and adherence. A patient attributing illness to spiritual causes may find pharmaceutical treatment insufficient without complementary spiritual healing (Napier et al., 2014).

**Communication patterns** vary across cultures regarding directness versus indirectness, appropriate question-asking, eye contact norms, personal space expectations, touch acceptability, emotional expression, and comfort with silence. Western medicine values direct communication and explicit information-sharing that may conflict with cultures preferring indirect communication and protecting individuals from difficult information (Galanti, 2015).

**Family structures and decision-making** differ regarding who constitutes family, gender roles and hierarchies, age-based authority, individual versus collective decision-making, and family involvement in health care. While Western bioethics prioritizes individual patient autonomy, many cultures emphasize family consensus and view protecting ill members from decision burdens as loving rather than paternalistic (Johnstone & Kanitsaki, 2009).

**Pain expression and management** shows cultural variation in pain reporting, emotional display during pain, medication acceptance versus tolerance preference, and meanings attributed to suffering. Some cultures view pain expression as weakness requiring stoicism, while others consider vocal expression appropriate. These differences affect pain assessment accuracy and treatment provision (Lasch, 2000).

**Death and dying practices** encompass beliefs about afterlife, appropriate death locations (home, hospital, hospice), information disclosure to dying individuals, life support decision-making, body handling, funeral traditions, and mourning durations. End-of-life care that ignores cultural practices may create distress and ethical conflicts (Searight & Gafford, 2005).

**Gender and modesty norms** influence acceptability of opposite-sex care providers, physical examination comfort, and discussion of sexual or reproductive health. Some cultures require same-sex providers for intimate care, while others prioritize provider expertise over gender. Health care systems that cannot accommodate these preferences create barriers and discomfort (Padela & del Pozo, 2011).

**Time orientation** varies between cultures emphasizing clock time and punctuality versus those valuing relational time and flexibility. Western medicine's strict appointment scheduling may conflict with cultures in which relationships take precedence over schedules, leading to missed appointments that providers misinterpret as noncompliance (Galanti, 2015).

## Implementing Culturally Humble Assessment and Intervention

Culturally responsive practice requires specific strategies that honor diversity while avoiding stereotyping. The following approaches integrate cultural humility into social work assessment and intervention:

**Start with open-ended cultural inquiry** rather than assumptions based on perceived ethnicity or cultural markers. Questions such as "What's important for me to understand about your cultural background?" "How does your family usually make health care decisions?" and "Are there cultural or religious practices we should know about?" invite patients to share relevant cultural information without imposing stereotypes. This approach recognizes that not all individuals identify strongly with ethnic cultures and that acculturation levels vary.

**Use the LEARN framework** (Berlin & Fowkes, 1983), a structured approach to cultural assessment and negotiation:

- **L**isten with sympathy and understanding to patient perspective.
- **E**xplain your perception of the situation and recommendations.
- **A**cknowledge and discuss differences and similarities.
- **R**ecommend treatment while incorporating patient perspective.
- **N**egotiate agreement that respects cultural values while ensuring safety.

This framework provides structure for navigating cultural differences without privileging medical perspectives or dismissing patient beliefs.

**Apply the Cultural Formulation Interview** from DSM-5, which assesses cultural identity, explanatory models of illness, psychosocial stressors, cultural features of the relationship with the clinician, and overall cultural assessment (American Psychiatric Association, 2013). While developed for psychiatric assessment, this framework applies broadly to medical social work, ensuring systematic attention to cultural dimensions.

**Attend to intersectionality** by recognizing that individuals hold multiple social identities (race, ethnicity, gender, sexual orientation, class, religion, disability, immigration status) that interact to shape experiences (Crenshaw, 1989). Culturally responsive practice acknowledges this complexity rather than reducing patients to single cultural categories. A Latina lesbian immigrant experiences health care differently than frameworks attending only to ethnicity would predict.

**Distinguish between cultural responsiveness and cultural stereotyping** by maintaining individual focus while acknowledging cultural patterns. Cultural knowledge provides hypotheses to explore, not assumptions to impose. The fact that some Asian cultures value family decision-making does not mean every Asian patient prefers this approach. Always ask individual preferences rather than assuming based on background.

**Address structural racism and historical trauma** that affects health and health care trust. Communities of color in the United States have experienced medical abuse including the Tuskegee Syphilis Study, forced sterilization, and ongoing discrimination. African Americans report higher medical mistrust, partly explained by historical and ongoing mistreatment (Hammond, 2010). Acknowledging this history and its impacts demonstrates respect and understanding.

**Partner with cultural brokers and community resources** including cultural liaisons, traditional healers, religious leaders, and community organizations. These partnerships enhance cultural understanding, build trust, and connect patients with culturally congruent support. Some health systems employ community health workers from specific cultural communities who provide navigation and interpretation.

## Language Access and Professional Interpretation

Language barriers significantly impair health care quality, contributing to medical errors, reduced satisfaction, poor comprehension, and health disparities (Karliner et al., 2007). Limited English proficiency (LEP) affects approximately 25 million people in the United States, with Spanish, Chinese, Vietnamese, and Korean representing the most common non-English languages (U.S. Census Bureau, 2019).

**Legal requirements** mandate language access in health care:

- **Title VI of the Civil Rights Act** prohibits discrimination based on national origin, interpreted to require language access for LEP individuals in federally funded programs, encompassing most health care settings (U.S. Department of Health and Human Services, 2003).
- **The Affordable Care Act** strengthened language access requirements, mandating that health plans provide interpretation and translated materials for common languages in service areas.
- **Joint Commission Standards** require organizations to identify patient language needs, provide interpretation, and translate key documents, with standards affecting accreditation status.

Despite legal requirements, language access implementation varies widely. Social workers must advocate for compliance while working within existing resources.

**Professional medical interpretation** improves communication accuracy, patient satisfaction, and clinical outcomes compared to ad hoc interpretation by family members or bilingual staff without interpreter training (Karliner et al., 2007). Professional interpreters receive training in medical terminology, ethics, cultural mediation, and interpretation technique. They function as neutral conduits maintaining confidentiality and accuracy.

**Interpretation modalities** include the following:

- **In-person interpretation** allows for nonverbal communication observation and provides fuller interaction. This proves ideal for complex conversations including mental health assessment, advance care planning, and family meetings. However, in-person interpreters may not be immediately available for all languages.
- **Telephone interpretation** provides quick access to numerous languages through interpretation services. Most hospitals maintain contracts with interpretation phone lines offering 24/7 access to hundreds of languages. While less ideal than in-person interpretation, phone services enable communication when in-person interpreters are unavailable.
- **Video remote interpretation (VRI)** combines telephone accessibility with visual component through tablets or computers. VRI enables observing nonverbal communication and documenting that professional interpretation occurred.

**Best practices for working with interpreters** include the following:

- **Position yourself and the interpreter appropriately.** Sit facing the patient with the interpreter to the side, maintaining eye contact with the patient rather than the interpreter.
- **Speak directly to the patient** using first-person language: "How are you feeling?" rather than "Ask her how she's feeling." This maintains the therapeutic relationship with the patient rather than the interpreter.

- **Use short sentences and pause frequently** to allow interpretation. Avoid long monologues that burden interpreter memory and may result in summarization rather than complete interpretation.
- **Speak at a moderate pace** without shouting. LEP does not mean hearing impairment. Speak clearly but naturally.
- **Avoid jargon, idioms, and metaphors** that may not translate. Use plain language: "heart attack" rather than "myocardial infarction," "feeling down" rather than "depressed affect."
- **Ask one question at a time** rather than compound questions that may confuse or result in partial answers.
- **Use teach-back method** to verify understanding: "Can you explain in your own words what we discussed?" This ensures accurate interpretation and comprehension.
- **Allow extra time** for interpreted encounters, typically 1.5–2 times the duration of English encounters, accounting for interpretation and cultural mediation.
- **Brief the interpreter beforehand** when possible, particularly for sensitive topics or complex information, allowing them to prepare and alerting them to content that may be culturally difficult.
- **Debrief with the interpreter afterward** to address any cultural concerns raised, clarify ambiguous responses, or process emotionally difficult content.

**What NOT to do:**

- **Never use family members as interpreters,** except in true emergencies when professional services are unavailable and delay would cause harm. Family interpretation creates confidentiality violations (what if patient doesn't want family to know certain information?), power imbalances (children translating for parents), distortion (family may filter or add information), and role confusion.
- **Do not use minor children as interpreters** under any circumstances. This violates childhood, exposes children to inappropriate medical information, creates role reversal, and may constitute neglect in some jurisdictions.
- **Avoid using bilingual staff without interpreter training** unless they have formal medical interpreter certification. Speaking a language does not qualify someone to interpret medical encounters requiring specialized knowledge and skills.

## Addressing Implicit Bias in Health Care

Implicit bias, unconscious attitudes and stereotypes affecting understanding and behavior, operates automatically outside conscious awareness (Greenwald & Banaji, 1995). Health care providers, including social workers, harbor implicit biases that affect clinical interactions despite explicit commitments to equality. Research demonstrates that even well-intentioned practitioners show implicit biases that correlate with disparities in pain management, treatment recommendations, and patient–provider communication (Hall et al., 2015).

### Common Implicit Biases in Health Care

1. **Racial bias:** Studies reveal that health care providers hold implicit preferences for White patients over Black patients and associate Black patients with noncompliance and decreased intelligence. These biases contribute to racial disparities in pain medication provision, cardiac care, and referrals to specialists (Green et al., 2007).
2. **Weight bias:** Health care providers view obese patients more negatively, attributing health problems to weight rather than exploring other causes, assuming lack of willpower and motivation, and providing less thorough care (Phelan et al., 2015).
3. **Socioeconomic bias:** Providers hold negative attitudes toward low-income patients, attributing

poverty to personal failings rather than structural factors, assuming lower health literacy and intelligence, and communicating less thoroughly (van Ryn & Burke, 2000).

4. **Substance use bias:** Patients with substance use disorders experience stigma and bias from health care providers who view addiction as moral failing, assume treatment-seeking manipulation, and provide less compassionate care (van Boekel et al., 2013).
5. **Disability bias:** Providers may unconsciously view lives with disabilities as less valuable, make assumptions about quality of life and treatment preferences, and communicate with caregivers rather than directly with patients who have disabilities (Iezzoni et al., 2021).

### Strategies to Address Implicit Bias

1. **Awareness and assessment:** Taking implicit association tests (available at implicit.harvard.edu) reveals unconscious biases. While awareness alone proves insufficient for change, it represents a necessary first step. Regular self-reflection about clinical interactions and decision-making identifies potential bias influences.
2. **Stereotype replacement:** When stereotypic thoughts arise, consciously replace them with non-stereotypic responses. Notice when making assumptions based on patient characteristics and intentionally generate alternative explanations (Devine et al., 2012).
3. **Counter-stereotypic imaging:** Regularly imagining counter-stereotypic examples (successful Black professionals, thin people with health problems, wealthy people needing assistance) weakens automatic stereotypic associations.
4. **Perspective-taking:** Imagining situations from patients' viewpoints and considering how their experiences differ from one's own reduces bias and increases empathy. This proves particularly important when patients' backgrounds differ significantly from providers'.
5. **Increased contact:** Meaningful contact with diverse populations under cooperative, equal-status conditions reduces prejudice and implicit bias (Pettigrew & Tropp, 2006). Diverse workforces and community partnerships create these opportunities.
6. **Mindfulness and slowing down:** Bias increases under time pressure and cognitive load when automatic processes dominate. Mindfulness practice and intentionally slowing decision-making in important situations reduce bias influence (Burgess et al., 2017).
7. **Accountability structures:** Awareness that clinical decisions will be reviewed or discussed with colleagues reduces bias. Consultation, supervision, and quality improvement processes create helpful accountability.
8. **Organizational commitment:** Individual efforts prove insufficient without institutional commitment to addressing disparities through policies, training, diverse workforce development, community partnerships, and systematic disparity monitoring.

## Cultural Humility as Ongoing Practice

Cultural humility represents a professional commitment rather than a competency checklist. This ongoing practice involves

- **continuous learning** through reading, training, community engagement, and learning from patients. Cultural dynamics evolve continuously; staying current requires intentional effort.
- **critical self-reflection** about one's own cultural identity, privileges, assumptions, and biases. Regular examination of how personal background shapes clinical perceptions maintains cultural awareness.
- **openness to correction** when cultural misunderstandings occur. Apologizing, adjusting approaches, and expressing appreciation for feedback demonstrates humility and builds trust.

- **advocacy for language access and cultural resources** within organizations, including interpretation services, diverse staff, culturally appropriate materials, and community partnerships.
- **humility about limits** by recognizing when cultural factors exceed your understanding and consulting cultural experts, community resources, or colleagues with relevant experience.

## Critical Thinking Questions

1. Analyze the shift from cultural competence to cultural humility through the lens of power relations in health care. How does each framework position patients and practitioners differently regarding authority and expertise? What implications does this have for truly patient-centered care?
2. Critique the concept of "culture" as it is typically used in health care literature. How might cultural frameworks essentialize and homogenize diverse populations? What theoretical alternatives might better capture the complexity of identity and social location?
3. Evaluate the evidence on implicit bias training effectiveness. What does research reveal about whether awareness-raising interventions actually change clinical behaviors and reduce disparities? What alternative or complementary approaches might prove more effective?
4. Examine language access through a health equity lens. How do language barriers exemplify broader patterns of structural inequality in health care? What would truly equitable language access require beyond interpretation services alone?

## Key Takeaways

- Cultural humility emphasizes lifelong learning, power-sharing, and institutional accountability rather than claiming cultural competence.
- Culture shapes health beliefs, communication patterns, family structures, pain expression, death practices, and health care interactions in profound ways.
- Culturally responsive assessment uses open-ended inquiry, frameworks such as LEARN and the Cultural Formulation Interview, and attention to intersectionality while avoiding stereotyping.
- Professional medical interpretation is legally required and clinically essential for quality care, with specific best practices for effective interpreter utilization.
- Implicit bias operates unconsciously but affects clinical interactions and contributes to health disparities, requiring individual and organizational strategies to address.
- Cultural humility represents ongoing ethical commitment requiring continuous learning, self-reflection, openness to correction, and advocacy for systemic change.

CHAPTER 9

# Mastering Discharge Planning

## Learning Objectives

By the end of this chapter, you will be able to do the following:

- Apply evidence-based discharge planning frameworks to reduce readmissions
- Assess social determinants of health affecting safe discharge
- Coordinate post-acute care services across health care and community systems
- Navigate insurance requirements and authorization processes
- Address health equity issues in discharge planning

## Discharge Planning as Core Social Work Function

Discharge planning, the process of preparing patients for transition from hospital to home or other care settings, represents a core medical social work function that significantly impacts patient outcomes, health care costs, and system efficiency. Effective discharge planning reduces hospital readmissions, improves patient satisfaction, facilitates recovery, and prevents adverse events during care transitions (Shepperd et al., 2013).

Despite its importance, discharge planning frequently occurs inadequately, characterized by rushed execution, poor coordination, insufficient patient and family preparation, and limited attention to social determinants of health. Approximately 20% of Medicare patients discharged from hospitals are readmitted within 30 days, many due to preventable factors including inadequate discharge planning (Jencks et al., 2009). These readmissions cost billions annually and represent quality failures.

Research consistently demonstrates social work's critical role in safe discharge. Studies link social work involvement to reduced readmissions, shorter lengths of stay, improved care coordination, better patient understanding of discharge instructions, and enhanced family preparedness (Coulton et al., 1982; Jack et al., 2009). Social workers' biopsychosocial perspective enables attention to medical needs alongside practical, emotional, and social factors affecting successful transitions.

The Patient Protection and Affordable Care Act increased discharge planning emphasis through readmission penalties for hospitals with excessive 30-day readmissions, creating financial incentives for improved discharge processes. Medicare's Hospital Readmissions Reduction Program reduces payments to hospitals with higher-than-expected readmissions for targeted conditions including heart failure, pneumonia, and joint replacement (Centers for Medicare & Medicaid Services, 2012). These policies position social workers as essential contributors to organizational quality and financial performance.

## Social Determinants of Health in Discharge Planning

Social determinants of health (SDOH), the conditions in which people are born, grow, live, work, and age, profoundly influence health outcomes and discharge safety (World Health Organization, 2008). Standard discharge planning focusing exclusively on medical factors while ignoring SDOH creates unsafe transitions for vulnerable populations.

**Key SDOH affecting discharge include**

1. **Housing stability and quality:** Homelessness or housing instability complicates discharge profoundly. How can someone recover from surgery without safe shelter? How can diabetic foot ulcers heal in unsanitary conditions? Beyond homelessness, housing quality matters. Third-floor walk-ups prove unsafe for patients with mobility impairments. Homes with mold or vermin exacerbate respiratory conditions. Unsafe neighborhoods create barriers to rehabilitation walks (Berkowitz et al., 2018).
2. **Food security:** Adequate nutrition proves essential for healing and chronic disease management. Food-insecure patients cannot maintain diabetic diets, heart-healthy eating, or renal restrictions. Medications should not be taken on empty stomachs when no food is available. Food insecurity affects medication adherence, emergency department use, and readmissions (Berkowitz et al., 2014).
3. **Transportation access:** Medical follow-up appointments, pharmacy visits, dialysis sessions, and rehabilitation services require reliable transportation. Patients without vehicles or public transit access miss appointments, leading to complications and readmissions. Transportation barriers disproportionately affect rural residents, elders, people with disabilities, and low-income individuals (Wallace et al., 2005).
4. **Social support and caregiving:** Recovery and chronic disease management often require caregiver assistance with medications, wound care, ambulation, and activities of daily living. Patients living alone without family or friends face dangerous isolation. Even when family exists, caregiver capacity varies based on employment, health, other responsibilities, and relationship quality. Caregiver burden and burnout affect care quality (Reinhard et al., 2008).
5. **Health literacy:** Understanding discharge instructions, medication regimens, warning signs requiring medical attention, and follow-up importance requires health literacy that many patients lack. Low health literacy correlates with poor outcomes, yet discharge teaching often occurs at inappropriate literacy levels using medical jargon (Berkman et al., 2011).
6. **Financial resources:** Out-of-pocket costs for medications, equipment, co-pays, and services create barriers. Cost-related medication non-adherence affects millions, increasing complications and readmissions. Financial strain influences whether patients can afford nutritious food, transportation, and home modifications (Sommers & Singh, 2021).
7. **Employment and insurance:** Job loss due to illness creates insurance loss, financial strain, and identity threats. Discharge planning must address insurance transitions, disability applications, and workplace accommodations for employed patients returning to work.

Comprehensive discharge planning systematically assesses these social determinants rather than discovering barriers at discharge when interventions prove difficult. Early SDOH screening enables proactive problem-solving and resource mobilization.

## Evidence-Based Discharge Planning Models

Several evidence-based models guide effective discharge planning, each emphasizing early initiation, patient and family engagement, and post-discharge follow-up.

**The Care Transitions Intervention (CTI)** developed by Coleman et al. (2006) emphasizes patient and caregiver activation through four pillars:

- medication self-management
- patient-centered record maintenance
- primary care and specialist follow-up
- knowledge of warning signs and when to seek help

CTI includes a transitions coach, often a nurse or social worker, who visits patients in hospital, attends discharge, makes home visits, and provides phone support for 30 days. Research demonstrates that CTI reduces readmissions and costs while improving patient satisfaction (Coleman et al., 2006).

**Project RED (re-engineered discharge)** provides a comprehensive toolkit that includes the following:

- Ascertain need for and obtain language interpreter.
- Make follow-up appointments before discharge.
- Plan for follow-up of test results.
- Organize post-discharge services.
- Identify correct medications and plan for patient to obtain them.
- Reconcile discharge plan with national guidelines.
- Teach written discharge plan to patient.
- Educate patient about diagnosis, medications, and warning signs.
- Assess patient understanding using teach-back.
- Provide contact information for questions.
- Expedite transmission of discharge summary to outpatient providers.

Project RED implementation significantly reduces readmissions and emergency department visits (Jack et al., 2009). The model's strength lies in systematic attention to multiple discharge components rather than assuming any single intervention suffices.

**Transitional care model (TCM)** focuses on high-risk older adults with complex needs, providing advanced practice nurse (often working with social workers) support through hospital visits, discharge accompaniment, home visits, and phone availability for six weeks post-discharge. TCM emphasizes comprehensive assessment, care plan development, coordination with physicians, and patient and caregiver education. Studies show reduced readmissions, improved satisfaction, and cost savings (Naylor et al., 2009).

**Common elements across evidence-based models** include

- early discharge planning initiation upon admission
- comprehensive assessment of medical and psychosocial needs
- patient and family education using teach-back
- medication reconciliation and education
- post-discharge follow-up appointments scheduled before discharge
- care coordination with outpatient providers
- post-discharge contact and support
- atention to SDOH and barriers

These models shift discharge planning from last-minute crisis management to proactive process beginning at admission and continuing post-discharge.

# Post-Acute Care Continuum and Levels of Care

Understanding various post-acute care settings and their admission criteria enables appropriate discharge planning matched to patient needs. Medicare and Medicaid establish specific coverage criteria social workers must navigate.

**Home with home health services** suits patients who are homebound but medically stable enough for intermittent skilled nursing or therapy rather than 24-hour care. **Medicare home health requirements** include physician certification of homebound status, a need for skilled nursing or therapy (not just custodial care), part-time or intermittent service needs, and a physician-ordered care plan. Patients must be medically stable but require skilled intervention. Services include skilled nursing, physical therapy, occupational therapy, speech therapy, home health aides, medical social work, and durable medical equipment (Centers for Medicare & Medicaid Services, 2023).

**Homebound status** requires that leaving home takes considerable effort due to a medical condition. Patients may leave home for medical appointments, religious services, and occasional short outings without losing homebound status. Confusion about homebound criteria often delays appropriate home health referrals.

**Inpatient rehabilitation facilities (IRFs)** provide intensive rehabilitation for patients who can tolerate and benefit from at least three hours of therapy daily. IRF-appropriate conditions include stroke, brain injury, spinal cord injury, amputation, hip fracture, and other traumatic injuries or complex medical conditions. **Medicare IRF requirements** include physician certification that intensive rehabilitation is needed, tolerance of three hours therapy daily, 24-hour rehabilitation nursing, and multidisciplinary team approach. Patients must demonstrate rehabilitation potential and motivation for intensive participation (Centers for Medicare & Medicaid Services, 2022).

**Long-term acute care hospitals (LTACHs)** serve medically complex patients requiring extended hospitalization, typically 25 days or longer. LTAC-appropriate patients often have multiple comorbidities, require ventilator weaning, have complex wounds, or need extended IV therapy. These facilities provide physician-directed care, complex medical management, and rehabilitation services for patients not yet stable for lower levels of care.

**Skilled nursing facilities (SNFs)** provide 24-hour skilled nursing and rehabilitation for patients requiring less-intensive services than IRFs or LTACHs. **Medicare SNF coverage requires** a three-day qualifying hospital stay (consecutive inpatient days, not including discharge day), admission to SNF within 30 days of hospital discharge, a need for skilled services daily (nursing or therapy), and physician certification that skilled care is needed. Medicare covers up to 100 days per benefit period (first 20 days fully covered, days 21–100 require copayment). After Medicare benefits exhaust, patients may self-pay or transition to Medicaid if eligible (Medicare.gov, 2023).

**The skilled versus custodial care** distinction proves critical. Medicare covers skilled care requiring professional expertise but not custodial care assistance with activities of daily living that any person could provide. This distinction sometimes creates coverage denials requiring appeals.

**Hospice care** serves patients with terminal illnesses and life expectancy of six months or less if the disease follows its expected course. Hospice provides comprehensive palliative care including nursing, physician services, medical equipment, medications related to terminal diagnosis, counseling, spiritual care, respite care, and bereavement services. Medicare hospice benefit covers these services with minimal out-of-pocket costs. Patients may elect hospice for two 90-day periods followed by unlimited 60-day periods with physician recertification (National Hospice and Palliative Care Organization, 2023).

**Barriers to hospice utilization** include prognostic uncertainty (physicians reluctant to state six-month prognosis), cultural values prioritizing life prolongation, misunderstanding hospice as "giving up," requirement to forgo curative treatment, and lack of awareness about hospice services.

## Navigating Insurance Authorization and Appeals

Understanding insurance requirements and authorization processes enables efficient discharge planning and reduces delays. Social workers often collaborate with case managers on insurance navigation, with social workers focusing on psychosocial assessment and resource coordination while case managers handle authorization logistics.

**Medicare Advantage Plans** (Medicare Part C) function as managed care, requiring prior authorization for post-acute services. These plans may have preferred provider networks, requiring patients to use specific facilities or requiring higher copayments for out-of-network care. Authorization denials require appeals with supporting documentation of medical necessity.

**Medicaid** requirements vary by state. Most states use managed care organizations for Medicaid beneficiaries, each with different authorization processes, networks, and covered services. Social workers must understand their state's Medicaid structure and individual patient's specific plan requirements.

**Private insurance** includes diverse plans with varying coverage. High-deductible health plans create significant out-of-pocket costs affecting service utilization. Some plans cover home health or rehabilitation poorly, limiting post-acute options. Prior authorization requirements vary, with some plans requiring authorization for home health, durable medical equipment, or post-acute facilities.

**Appeals Processes** exist when insurers deny coverage. Social workers support appeals in the following ways:

- documenting medical and psychosocial necessity thoroughly
- obtaining physician letters supporting need for services
- highlighting safety risks of denial
- utilizing hospital utilization review and case management resources
- connecting patients with insurance advocates or legal aid when needed
- knowing insurance appeal timelines and requirements

**Financial counseling and assistance programs** help patients facing costs. Hospitals employ financial counselors who identify charity care eligibility, payment plans, and medication assistance programs. Social workers connect patients to these resources and advocate for financial support.

## Addressing Health Equity in Discharge Planning

Discharge planning processes can perpetuate or mitigate health disparities. Research documents that marginalized populations experience worse discharge outcomes including higher readmissions, less access to post-acute services, and inadequate discharge support (Kind et al., 2014).

**Disparities in post-acute care access:** Studies show that Black and Hispanic patients receive less post-acute rehabilitation compared to White patients with similar medical needs, even controlling for insurance. Patients from disadvantaged zip codes face limited facility options and may be discharged home without adequate support due to placement barriers (Groeneveld et al., 2018).

**Language barriers in discharge teaching:** LEP patients receive less thorough discharge education, have lower comprehension of discharge instructions, and experience higher readmissions. Effective discharge planning requires professional interpretation and translated materials (Karliner et al., 2007).

**Health literacy disparities:** Low health literacy disproportionately affects older adults, racial and ethnic minorities, and low-income individuals. Standard discharge teaching often occurs at levels exceeding patients' health literacy, compromising safety (Berkman et al., 2011).

**Homelessness and housing instability:** Hospitals sometimes discharge patients experiencing homelessness to shelters or streets without addressing barriers to recovery. "Homeless discharges" represent profound failures of care, yet they occur regularly in many systems (Doran et al., 2013).

**Equity-oriented discharge planning** requires

- systematic SDOH screening for all patients
- addressing of barriers proactively rather than at discharge
- culturally responsive discharge education using professional interpretation
- health literacy–appropriate materials and teach-back methods
- community partnerships with organizations serving marginalized populations
- advocacy for patients facing placement discrimination
- protocols preventing unsafe discharges of unstably housed individuals
- data collection and analysis regarding discharge disparities
- organizational commitment to health equity

Social workers serve as health equity champions in discharge planning, naming injustices, advocating for individual patients, and pushing for systemic improvements.

## Practical Discharge Planning Skills

Beyond theoretical frameworks, effective discharge planning requires practical competencies.

**Comprehensive discharge assessment** begins at admission and explores the following:

- baseline functional status (ADLs, IADLs, mobility)
- living situation (housing type, accessibility, safety)
- social support and caregiver capacity
- financial resources and insurance coverage
- health literacy and comprehension
- transportation access
- food security and nutrition resources
- cultural preferences and practices
- barriers to follow-up care
- patient and family discharge preferences and goals

**Patient and family education** uses the teach-back method:

- Explain diagnosis and treatment plan in plain language.
- Review medications including purpose, timing, and side effects.
- Demonstrate and have patient/caregiver demonstrate wound care, medical equipment use, or other care tasks.
- Identify warning signs requiring medical attention.
- Ensure understanding of follow-up appointments and their importance.
- Provide written instructions appropriate to health literacy level.
- Use translation services and provide materials in primary language.

**Medication reconciliation** ensures accuracy:

- Compare pre-admission medications to hospital medications to discharge medications.
- Identify and clarify discrepancies with pharmacy and physicians.
- Ensure patient/family understands which medications to continue, discontinue, or start.
- Address medication costs and connect to assistance programs.
- Coordinate with discharge pharmacy or mail-order pharmacy.
- Provide medication list with names, dosages, purposes, and timing.

**Post-discharge follow-up coordination:**

- Schedule primary care and specialist appointments before discharge when possible.
- Provide appointment information in writing with date, time, location, and transportation details.
- Confirm that outpatient providers received discharge summary.
- Arrange home health or other services to begin promptly after discharge.
- Provide contact information for questions or concerns.
- Make follow-up phone calls post-discharge to assess adjustment and address problems.

**Documentation** creates a comprehensive discharge record:

- psychosocial assessment findings
- discharge barriers identified and addressed
- family meetings and education provided
- services arranged and referrals made
- patient and family understanding and preparedness
- remaining concerns and follow-up needed
- communication with outpatient providers

## Critical Thinking Questions

1. Analyze discharge planning through a critical political economy lens. How do hospital financial incentives (diagnosis-related group payments, readmission penalties) shape discharge practices in ways that may conflict with patient needs? What structural changes would better align institutional and patient interests?
2. Examine the concept of "medical necessity" as it operates in insurance authorization. How does the construction of medical necessity privilege biomedical factors while marginalizing social determinants of health? What advocacy strategies might challenge narrow necessity definitions?
3. Evaluate the ethics of discharging patients experiencing homelessness to shelters or streets. What ethical principles does this practice violate? What institutional and structural changes would be required to eliminate unsafe homeless discharges? What role should social workers play in challenging these practices?
4. Critique the assumption underlying most discharge planning models that patients have access to stable housing, reliable caregiving, adequate finances, and other resources. How might discharge planning frameworks be redesigned to center the realities of multiply marginalized populations?

## Key Takeaways

- Evidence-based discharge planning reduces readmissions, improves outcomes, and proves cost-effective through early initiation, comprehensive assessment, patient education using teach-back, and post-discharge follow-up.
- Social determinants of health including housing, food security, transportation, social support, health literacy, and financial resources profoundly affect discharge safety and must be systematically assessed.
- Post-acute care continuum includes home health, inpatient rehabilitation, long-term acute care, skilled nursing, and hospice, each with specific admission criteria and insurance coverage requirements.
- Insurance navigation requires understanding Medicare, Medicaid, and private insurance authorization processes, coverage criteria, and appeals options.

- Health equity in discharge planning demands attention to disparities, culturally responsive education, SDOH-focused intervention, and advocacy against discriminatory practices.
- Effective discharge planning combines systematic assessment, patient-centered education, care coordination, and documentation.

CHAPTER 10

# Educating About Advance Directives

## Learning Objectives

By the end of this chapter, you will be able to do the following:

- Explain legal and ethical foundations for advance care planning
- Facilitate conversations about end-of-life preferences using evidence-based communication strategies
- Navigate common barriers to advance directive completion across diverse populations
- Distinguish between various advance directive documents and their applications
- Address cultural and spiritual dimensions of advance care planning

## Legal and Ethical Foundations of Advance Care Planning

Advance care planning (ACP) enables individuals to articulate preferences for medical treatment in scenarios where they may lose decision-making capacity, ensuring that care aligns with their values and goals rather than medical defaults or family assumptions (Sudore & Fried, 2010). Advance directives, the legal documents recording these preferences, emerged from bioethical principles emphasizing patient autonomy and informed consent.

**The Patient Self-Determination Act of 1990** (PSDA) represented landmark legislation requiring Medicare- and Medicaid-participating institutions to inform patients about their rights to accept or refuse treatment and to execute advance directives. The PSDA mandates that hospitals, nursing homes, home health agencies, hospices, and health maintenance organizations provide written information about advance directives upon admission, document whether patients have directives, and educate staff and community about advance care planning (U.S. Department of Health and Human Services, 1991).

Despite PSDA implementation over 30 years ago, advance directive completion rates remain low. National studies show that only 30%–40% of adults have advance directives, with even lower rates among younger adults and racial and ethnic minorities (Yadav et al., 2017). This implementation gap reflects multiple factors including discomfort discussing death, lack of awareness about advance directives, difficulty imagining future health states, mistrust of health care systems, and inadequate physician-patient communication about goals of care (Schicktanz et al., 2009).

**Ethical principles** supporting advance care planning include the following.

**Autonomy** respects individuals' rights to make decisions about their own medical care, including refusing life-sustaining treatment. Advance directives extend autonomy to situations where illness or injury prevents contemporaneous decision-making.

**Beneficence and non-maleficence** obligate health care providers to act in patients' best interests while avoiding harm. When patients cannot communicate, advance directives guide providers regarding what patients consider beneficial versus harmful, preventing unwanted aggressive interventions or premature treatment withdrawal.

**Respect for persons** recognizes intrinsic human dignity and requires treating individuals as autonomous agents. Advance care planning honors personhood by ensuring that medical treatment reflects individuals' values even when they cannot speak.

**Justice** requires fair distribution of health care resources and non-discrimination in access to advance care planning support. Disparities in advance directive completion and quality conversations represent justice failures requiring attention.

## Types of Advance Directives and Legal Documents

Multiple legal documents comprise comprehensive advance care planning. Understanding each document's purpose and limitations enables effective patient education:

**A Living Will** articulates preferences regarding life-sustaining treatments (mechanical ventilation, cardiopulmonary resuscitation, artificial nutrition and hydration, dialysis) typically in scenarios of terminal illness, permanent unconsciousness, or advanced dementia. Living wills address treatment preferences but do not designate decision-makers. Limitations include difficulty anticipating all scenarios, vague language open to interpretation, and lack of flexibility as circumstances change (Fagerlin & Schneider, 2004).

**Medical Power of Attorney** (Health Care Proxy, Health Care Agent, Durable Power of Attorney for Health Care) designates a trusted person to make medical decisions if the individual loses capacity. This proves more flexible than living wills because the designated agent can interpret preferences in specific situations rather than attempting to anticipate every possibility. Agents should understand the person's values, communicate effectively with medical teams, and make decisions the person would make, not what the agent prefers (Sabatino, 2010).

**Do Not Resuscitate (DNR) Orders** instruct health care providers not to perform CPR if cardiac or respiratory arrest occurs. Hospital DNR orders apply within the facility. **Out-of-hospital DNR orders** (also called DNR Comfort Care, POLST, MOLST) instruct emergency medical services not to initiate resuscitation. These orders require physician signatures and should be readily visible (often on brightly colored paper displayed on refrigerators). Without out-of-hospital DNR orders, emergency personnel must attempt resuscitation regardless of living will statements.

**Physician Orders for Life-Sustaining Treatment (POLST) / Medical Orders for Life-Sustaining Treatment (MOLST)** represent medical orders, not advance directives, completing alongside advance directives for seriously ill patients. POLST/MOLST forms, signed by physicians, specify medical orders regarding CPR, medical interventions (comfort measures only, limited interventions, full treatment), antibiotics, and artificial nutrition. Unlike advance directives that activate only when patients lose capacity, POLST forms constitute current medical orders implemented immediately. These forms suit patients with advanced illness or frailty but not healthy individuals planning for distant future scenarios (Hickman et al., 2010).

**Importance of surrogate decision-maker designation:** When patients lack advance directives and lose capacity, states follow default surrogate hierarchies (typically spouse, adult children, parents, siblings). These defaults may not align with patients' preferences. Designating health care agents through medical power of attorney ensures that the person most trusted makes decisions, whether or not they are family. This proves particularly critical for unmarried partners, chosen family, LGBTQ+ individuals, and others whose important relationships may not be recognized through default hierarchies.

## Evidence-Based Advance Care Planning Communication

Research reveals that advance care planning conversations, when conducted skillfully, improve outcomes including increased completion of advance directives, greater concordance between preferences and care received, reduced unwanted intensive care, increased hospice utilization, better quality of life at end of life, and reduced family decisional conflict and post-death distress (Brinkman-Stoppelenburg et al., 2014).

However, conversations conducted poorly or avoided entirely contribute to aggressive end-of-life care that patients may not want, family guilt about decisions made, moral distress among health care professionals required to provide treatments they believe are harmful, and wasted health care resources.

**Barriers to advance care planning conversations** include

**Patient and family barriers:**

- fear that discussing death tempts fate or accelerates dying
- cultural or religious prohibitions against death discussion
- difficulty imagining future health states
- uncertainty about preferences
- distrust of health care system
- belief that family knows preferences without documentation
- avoidance of emotionally difficult topics

**Health care provider barriers:**

- discomfort discussing death
- lack of training in communication skills
- perception of inadequate time
- concern about removing hope
- uncertainty about when to initiate conversations
- fear of emotional reactions
- billing and reimbursement confusion

**Systematic barriers:**

- Fragmented health care without relationship continuity
- Acute care focus rather than long-term planning
- Lack of standardized processes
- Inadequate interdisciplinary collaboration
- Missing interpretation services for LEP patients

**The Respecting Choices model** provides evidence-based framework for advance care planning conversations with patients and surrogates, emphasizing trained facilitators (often social workers), systematic introduction of conversations, structured conversation guides, and documentation (Hammes et al., 2010). Research demonstrates increased advance directive completion, improved satisfaction, and reduced unwanted intensive care in systems implementing Respecting Choices.

**Communication strategies for advance care planning:**

1. **Introduce the topic normalized and early:** Frame advance care planning as routine health care for all adults, not crisis intervention for dying patients. "I talk with all my patients about advance care planning to ensure we understand your health care preferences. Could we spend some time discussing this today?" This approach reduces death anxiety and stigma.

2. **Explore values and goals before specific treatments:** Rather than beginning with "Do you want CPR?" explore broader values: What's most important to you in your health care? What are you hoping for? What are you worried about? How much are you willing to go through for possible benefits? Understanding values enables later treatment decisions consistent with those values (Sudore et al., 2017).
3. **Use "wish" language:** "If you became seriously ill and couldn't speak for yourself, would you wish to have all possible life support even if doctors thought it unlikely to help, or would you wish to focus on comfort?"
   "What would you wish your loved ones to know about your preferences?" This language feels less threatening than directive medical language.
4. **Address common misconceptions:** Many people misunderstand CPR effectiveness, believing television portrayals showing young, healthy people surviving. Educate that CPR succeeds in perhaps 15%–20% of hospitalized patients, lower outside hospitals, with meaningful recovery much rarer in patients with serious underlying illness (Girotra et al., 2012). This information enables informed decisions.
5. **Support decision-maker preparation:** Help designated health care agents understand their role: "Your job is to make the decisions your mother would make if she could tell us herself, based on what she values, not what you prefer for her." Prepare for difficult decisions and provide permission to follow loved ones' wishes even when emotionally hard.
6. **Document thoroughly:** Record conversations, preferences expressed, designated agents, and patients' understanding in medical records. Ensure advance directive documents are uploaded to electronic health records and that outpatient providers receive copies.
7. **Revisit periodically:** Preferences change as health status changes. Encourage updating advance directives after major health events, at regular intervals (annually or every few years), and when life circumstances change (marriage, divorce, birth of children).
8. **Advance care planning across the lifespan:** While advance directives prove most relevant for older adults and those with serious illness, conversations with younger, healthy adults about values and general preferences plant seeds for later detailed planning. These early conversations reduce avoidance and normalize planning.

## Cultural and Spiritual Dimensions of Advance Care Planning

Cultural and spiritual beliefs profoundly shape attitudes toward advance care planning, death discussion, medical decision-making, and appropriate care at end of life. Culturally responsive advance care planning requires understanding diverse perspectives without imposing dominant culture values (Johnstone & Kanitsaki, 2009).

### Individualism Versus Collectivism

Western bioethics emphasizes individual patient autonomy in advance care planning. Many non-Western cultures prioritize family or community decision-making, viewing individual advance directives as inappropriate autonomy assertion that excludes family. Some families prefer not to burden seriously ill members with decisions, making choices collectively to protect patients. Culturally responsive practice respects these preferences rather than insisting on Western autonomy models (Blackhall et al., 1995).

## Truth-Telling and Prognostic Disclosure

Some cultures value direct, explicit death discussion, while others consider such conversations harmful, inappropriate, or disrespectful. Families may request that patients not be told terminal prognoses, believing knowledge would accelerate death or destroy hope. These situations create ethical tensions between respect for cultural values and Western informed consent principles. Approaches respecting both autonomy and culture include asking patients their preferences for information and including family in conversations when patients desire (Searight & Gafford, 2005).

## Fate, Divine Will, and Human Control

Religious and spiritual beliefs influence whether individuals view life-death decisions as appropriate human choices or matters of divine will. Some believe that God alone determines life and death, making treatment limitation decisions presumptuous. Others view medical technology as interfering with natural dying that should be accepted. These beliefs deserve respect in advance care planning conversations, exploring how medical treatments align with spiritual values (Puchalski et al., 2009).

## Distrust and Historical Trauma

African Americans and other marginalized communities experience medical mistrust rooted in historical abuses including the Tuskegee Syphilis Study, forced sterilization, experimentation without consent, and ongoing discrimination. This mistrust extends to advance directives, with concerns that DNR orders lead to premature treatment cessation or inferior care. Culturally competent conversations acknowledge this history, address concerns transparently, and build trust through relationship rather than dismissing fears as unfounded (Crawley et al., 2000).

## Diverse Afterlife Beliefs

Beliefs about what follows death shape end-of-life preferences. Those believing in heaven may view death as transition to better existence, affecting treatment preferences. Reincarnation beliefs create different perspectives. Those viewing death as nonexistence may emphasize life prolongation differently. Advance care planning conversations benefit from exploring these beliefs and their treatment implications (Puchalski et al., 2009).

## Culturally Responsive Strategies

- Begin with open questions about cultural and spiritual beliefs affecting health care.
- Avoid assumptions based on perceived ethnicity or religion.
- Partner with chaplains, cultural liaisons, or community religious leaders.
- Offer family involvement in conversations when patients prefer.
- Provide advance directive education respecting diverse decision-making models.
- Use professional interpretation and translated materials.
- Create advance directives flexible enough to honor cultural values.
- Document cultural preferences and beliefs informing care preferences.

# Advance Care Planning for Specific Populations

Certain populations require tailored advance care planning approaches:

1. **Patients with dementia:** Early-stage dementia represents crucial time for advance care planning while capacity remains. Conversations should address preferences for treatment intensity, feeding

tube wishes, acceptable quality of life, and preferred care locations. As dementia progresses, surrogate decision-makers rely heavily on these earlier conversations (Dening et al., 2011).

2. **Pediatric advance care planning:** Children with life-limiting conditions benefit from advance care planning involving parents and, when developmentally appropriate, children themselves. Approaches differ from adult planning, emphasizing family decision-making and developmentally appropriate child involvement (Lyon et al., 2014).
3. **Individuals with intellectual/developmental disabilities:** This population historically lacked access to advance care planning, with decisions defaulting to guardians or family. Supported decision-making models enable individuals with I/DD to participate meaningfully in advance care planning, with appropriate communication supports and decision-making assistance (Arstein-Kerslake et al., 2017).
4. **LGBTQ+ individuals:** This population faces unique challenges including partners not recognized through default surrogate hierarchies, family rejection creating decision-making conflicts, and past discrimination creating health care mistrust. Advance care planning proves particularly important for designating chosen family as decision-makers and articulating wishes explicitly (Stein et al., 2020).

## Critical Thinking Questions

1. Analyze the Patient Self-Determination Act through a critical lens. While intended to promote autonomy, how might mandated advance directive discussions inadvertently coerce vulnerable patients or reflect dominant culture values about death and autonomy? What alternative approaches might better honor diverse perspectives?
2. Evaluate the assumption underlying advance care planning that individuals can and should make binding future decisions about hypothetical health states. What does research reveal about the stability of preferences over time? How do anticipated and actual preferences differ in studies of seriously ill patients? What implications does this have for advance directive validity?
3. Examine advance care planning disparities through an intersectional framework. How do race, class, education, and other social locations interact to shape advance directive completion and quality? What structural changes would address root causes of these disparities rather than individualizing the problem?
4. Critique the concept of "medical futility" as it operates in end-of-life decision-making. How might futility determinations reflect physician values and biases rather than objective medical judgments? Who should hold authority to determine futility, and what role should advance directives play in these conflicts?

## Key Takeaways

- The Patient Self-Determination Act of 1990 mandates advance care planning education, yet completion rates remain low due to multiple patient, provider, and system barriers.
- Comprehensive advance care planning includes living wills, medical power of attorney, DNR orders, and POLST/MOLST forms, each serving distinct purposes.
- Evidence-based communication strategies emphasize values clarification, normalized early conversations, addressing misconceptions, and preparing surrogate decision-makers.
- Cultural and spiritual beliefs profoundly shape advance care planning attitudes, requiring culturally responsive approaches that honor diverse decision-making models.
- Special populations including patients with dementia, children with life-limiting conditions, individuals with disabilities, and LGBTQ+ individuals require tailored advance care planning support.

- Social workers play essential roles in facilitating advance care planning conversations, addressing barriers, and ensuring culturally appropriate approaches.

# Section II References


American Psychiatric Association. (2013). *Diagnostic and statistical manual of mental disorders* (5th ed.). https://doi.org/10.1176/appi.books.9780890425596

Arstein-Kerslake, A., Gooding, P., Andrews, J., & McSherry, B. (2017). Human rights and supported decision-making for people with intellectual disability. *Journal of Intellectual & Developmental Disability, 42*(3), 285–291. https://doi.org/10.1177/10442073211026332

Beder, J. (2006). *Hospital social work: The interface of medicine and caring*. Routledge.

Berkman, N. D., Sheridan, S. L., Donahue, K. E., Halpern, D. J., & Crotty, K. (2011). Low health literacy and health outcomes: An updated systematic review. *Annals of Internal Medicine, 155*(2), 97–107. https://doi.org/10.7326/0003-4819-155-2-201107190-00005

Berkowitz, S. A., Hulberg, A. C., Standish, S., Reznor, G., & Atlas, S. J. (2017). Addressing unmet basic resource needs as part of chronic cardiometabolic disease management. *JAMA Internal Medicine, 177*(2), 244–252. https://doi.org/10.1001/jamainternmed.2016.7691

Berkowitz, S. A., Seligman, H. K., Rigdon, J., Meigs, J. B., & Basu, S. (2018). Supplemental Nutrition Assistance Program participation and health care use: A systematic review. *Health Affairs, 37*(4), 577–585. https://doi.org/10.1377/hlthaff.2017.1371

Berlin, E. A., & Fowkes, W. C. (1983). A teaching framework for cross-cultural health care. *Western Journal of Medicine, 139*(6), 934–938.

Betancourt, J. R., Green, A. R., Carrillo, J. E., & Ananeh-Firempong, O. (2003). Defining cultural competence: A practical framework for addressing racial/ethnic disparities in health and health care. *Public Health Reports, 118*(4), 293–302. https://doi.org/10.1016/S0033-3549(04)50253-4

Blackhall, L. J., Murphy, S. T., Frank, G., Michel, V., & Azen, S. (1995). Ethnicity and attitudes toward patient autonomy. *JAMA, 274*(10), 820–825. https://doi.org/10.1001/jama.1995.03530100060035

Boss, P. (2011). *Loving someone who has dementia: How to find hope while coping with stress and grief*. Jossey-Bass.

Brinkman-Stoppelenburg, A., Rietjens, J. A., & van der Heide, A. (2014). The effects of advance care planning on end-of-life care: A systematic review. *Palliative Medicine, 28*(8), 1000–1025. https://doi.org/10.1177/0269216314526272

Brymer, M., Jacobs, A., Layne, C., Pynoos, R., Ruzek, J., Steinberg, A., Vernberg, E., & Watson, P. (2006). *Psychological first aid: Field operations guide* (2nd ed.). National Child Traumatic Stress Network and National Center for PTSD.

Burgess, D. J., Beach, M. C., & Saha, S. (2017). Mindfulness practice: A promising approach to reducing the effects of clinician implicit bias on patients. *Patient Education and Counseling, 100*(2), 372–376. https://doi.org/10.1016/j.pec.2016.09.005

Caplan, G. (1964). *Principles of preventive psychiatry*. Basic Books.

Centers for Medicare & Medicaid Services. (2012). *Readmissions Reduction Program*. https://www.cms.gov/Medicare/medicare-fee-for-service-payment/acuteinpatientPPS/readmissions-reduction-program

Centers for Medicare & Medicaid Services. (2022). *Inpatient rehabilitation facility prospective payment system*. https://www.cms.gov/medicare/payment/prospective-payment-systems/inpatient-rehabilitation

Centers for Medicare & Medicaid Services. (2023). *Home health prospective payment system*. https://www.cms.gov/Medicare/Medicare-Fee-for-Service-Payment/HomeHealthPPS

Coleman, E. A., Parry, C., Chalmers, S., & Min, S. J. (2006). The care transitions intervention: Results of a randomized controlled trial. *Archives of Internal Medicine, 166*(17), 1822–1828. https://doi.org/10.1001/archinte.166.17.1822

Coulton, C. J., Dunkle, R. E., Goode, R. A., & MacKintosh, J. (1982). Discharge planning and decision making. *Health & Social Work, 7*(4), 253–261. https://doi.org/10.1093/hsw/7.4.253

Crawley, L., Payne, R., Bolden, J., Payne, T., Washington, P., & Williams, S. (2000). Palliative and end-of-life care in the African American community. *JAMA, 284*(19), 2518–2521. https://doi.org/10.1001/jama.284.19.2518

Crenshaw, K. (1989). Demarginalizing the intersection of race and sex: A Black feminist critique of antidiscrimination doctrine, feminist theory and antiracist politics. *University of Chicago Legal Forum, 1989*(1), 139–167.

Dening, K. H., Jones, L., & Sampson, E. L. (2011). Advance care planning for people with dementia: A review. *International Psychogeriatrics, 23*(10), 1535–1551. https://doi.org/10.1017/S1041610211001608

Devine, P. G., Forscher, P. S., Austin, A. J., & Cox, W. T. (2012). Long-term reduction in implicit race bias: A prejudice habit-breaking intervention. *Journal of Experimental Social Psychology, 48*(6), 1267–1278. https://doi.org/10.1016/j.jesp.2012.06.003

Doka, K. J. (Ed.). (2002). *Disenfranchised grief: New directions, challenges, and strategies for practice*. Research Press.

Doran, K. M., Ragins, K. T., Iacomacci, A. L., Cunningham, A., Jubanyik, K. J., & Jenq, G. Y. (2013). The revolving hospital door: Hospital readmissions among patients who are homeless. *Medical Care, 51*(9), 767–773. https://doi.org/10.1097/MLR.0b013e31829fafbb

Fagerlin, A., & Schneider, C. E. (2004). Enough: The failure of the living will. *Hastings Center Report, 34*(2), 30–42. https://doi.org/10.2307/3528252

Figley, C. R. (Ed.). (1995). *Compassion fatigue: Coping with secondary traumatic stress disorder in those who treat the traumatized*. Brunner/Mazel.

Foronda, C., Baptiste, D. L., Reinholdt, M. M., & Ousman, K. (2016). Cultural humility: A concept analysis. *Journal of Transcultural Nursing, 27*(3), 210–217. https://doi.org/10.1177/1043659615592677

Galanti, G. A. (2015). *Caring for patients from different cultures* (5th ed.). University of Pennsylvania Press.

Girotra, S., Nallamothu, B. K., Spertus, J. A., Li, Y., Krumholz, H. M., & Chan, P. S. (2012). Trends in survival after in-hospital cardiac arrest. *New England Journal of Medicine, 367*(20), 1912–1920. https://doi.org/10.1056/NEJMoa1109148

Green, A. R., Carney, D. R., Pallin, D. J., Ngo, L. H., Raymond, K. L., Iezzoni, L. I., & Banaji, M. R. (2007). Implicit bias among physicians and its prediction of thrombolysis decisions for Black and White patients. *Journal of General Internal Medicine, 22*(9), 1231–1238. https://doi.org/10.1007/s11606-007-0258-5

Greenwald, A. G., & Banaji, M. R. (1995). Implicit social cognition: Attitudes, self-esteem, and stereotypes. *Psychological Review, 102*(1), 4–27. https://doi.org/10.1037/0033-295X.102.1.4

Groeneveld, P. W., Laufer, S. B., & Garber, A. M. (2005). Technology diffusion, hospital variation, and racial disparities among elderly Medicare beneficiaries: 1989-2000. *Medical Care, 43*(4), 320–329. https://doi.org/10.1097/01.mlr.0000156849.15166.ec

Hall, W. J., Chapman, M. V., Lee, K. M., Merino, Y. M., Thomas, T. W., Payne, B. K., Eng, E., Day, S. H., & Coyne-Beasley, T. (2015). Implicit racial/ethnic bias among health care professionals and its influence on health care outcomes: A systematic review. *American Journal of Public Health, 105*(12), e60–e76. https://doi.org/10.2105/AJPH.2015.302903

Hammes, B. J., Rooney, B. L., & Gundrum, J. D. (2010). A comparative, retrospective, observational study of the prevalence, availability, and specificity of advance care plans in a county that implemented an advance care planning microsystem. *Journal of the American Geriatrics Society, 58*(7), 1249–1255. https://doi.org/10.1111/j.1532-5415.2010.02956.x

Hammond, W. P. (2010). Psychosocial correlates of medical mistrust among African American men. *American Journal of Community Psychology, 45*(1–2), 87–106. https://doi.org/10.1007/s10464-009-9280-6

Hickman, S. E., Nelson, C. A., Perrin, N. A., Moss, A. H., Hammes, B. J., & Tolle, S. W. (2010). A comparison of methods to communicate treatment preferences in nursing facilities: Traditional practices versus the physician orders for life-sustaining treatment program. *Journal of the American Geriatrics Society, 58*(7), 1241–1248. https://doi.org/10.1111/j.1532-5415.2010.02955.x

Holley, C. K., & Mast, B. T. (2009). The impact of anticipatory grief on caregiver burden in dementia caregivers. *The Gerontologist, 49*(3), 388–396. https://doi.org/10.1093/geront/gnp061

Hook, J. N., Davis, D. E., Owen, J., Worthington, E. L., & Utsey, S. O. (2013). Cultural humility: Measuring openness to culturally diverse clients. *Journal of Counseling Psychology, 60*(3), 353–366. https://doi.org/10.1037/a0032595

Iezzoni, L. I., Rao, S. R., Ressalam, J., Bolcic-Jankovic, D., Agaronnik, N. D., Donelan, K., Lagu, T., & Campbell, E. G. (2021). Physicians' perceptions of people with disability and their health care. *Health Affairs, 40*(2), 297–306. https://doi.org/10.1377/hlthaff.2020.01452

Institute of Medicine. (2001). *Crossing the quality chasm: A new health system for the 21st century*. National Academies Press.

Institute of Medicine. (2003). *Unequal treatment: Confronting racial and ethnic disparities in health care*. National Academies Press.

Jack, B. W., Chetty, V. K., Anthony, D., Greenwald, J. L., Sanchez, G. M., Johnson, A. E., Forsythe, S. R., O'Donnell, J. K., Paasche-Orlow, M. K., Manasseh, C., Martin, S., & Culpepper, L. (2009). A reengineered hospital discharge program to decrease rehospitalization: A randomized trial. *Annals of Internal Medicine, 150*(3), 178–187. https://doi.org/10.7326/0003-4819-150-3-200902030-00007

James, R. K., & Gilliland, B. E. (2017). *Crisis intervention strategies* (8th ed.). Cengage Learning.

Jencks, S. F., Williams, M. V., & Coleman, E. A. (2009). Rehospitalizations among patients in the Medicare fee-for-service program. *New England Journal of Medicine, 360*(14), 1418–1428. https://doi.org/10.1056/NEJMsa0803563

Johnstone, M. J., & Kanitsaki, O. (2009). Ethics and advance care planning in a culturally diverse society. *Journal of Transcultural Nursing, 20*(4), 405–416. https://doi.org/10.1177/1043659609340803

Kanel, K. (2019). *A guide to crisis intervention* (6th ed.). Cengage Learning.

Karliner, L. S., Jacobs, E. A., Chen, A. H., & Mutha, S. (2007). Do professional interpreters improve clinical care for patients with limited English proficiency? A systematic review of the literature. *Health Services Research, 42*(2), 727–754. https://doi.org/10.1111/j.1475-6773.2006.00629.x

Keall, R. M., Clayton, J. M., & Butow, P. N. (2015). Therapeutic life review in palliative care: A systematic review of quantitative evaluations. *Journal of Pain and Symptom Management, 49*(4), 747–761. https://doi.org/10.1016/j.jpainsymman.2014.08.015

Kind, A. J., Jencks, S., Brock, J., Yu, M., Bartels, C., Ehlenbach, W., Greenberg, C., & Smith, M. (2014). Neighborhood socioeconomic disadvantage and 30-day rehospitalization: A retrospective cohort study. *Annals of Internal Medicine, 161*(11), 765–774. https://doi.org/10.7326/M13-2946

Klass, D., Silverman, P. R., & Nickman, S. L. (Eds.). (1996). *Continuing bonds: New understandings of grief.* Taylor & Francis.

Kleespies, P. M. (Ed.). (2009). *Behavioral emergencies: An evidence-based resource for evaluating and managing risk of suicide, violence, and victimization*. American Psychological Association.

Kleinman, A., & Benson, P. (2006). Anthropology in the clinic: The problem of cultural competency and how to fix it. *PLoS Medicine, 3*(10), e294. https://doi.org/10.1371/journal.pmed.0030294

Kramer, B. J., Kavanaugh, M., Trentham-Dietz, A., Walsh, M., & Yonker, J. A. (2010). Predictors of family conflict at the end of life: The experience of spouses and adult children of persons with lung cancer. *The Gerontologist, 50*(2), 215–225. https://doi.org/10.1093/geront/gnp121

Kübler-Ross, E. (1969). *On death and dying*. Macmillan.

Kübler-Ross, E., & Kessler, D. (2005). *On grief and grieving: Finding the meaning of grief through the five stages of loss.* Scribner.

Lasch, K. E. (2000). Culture, pain, and culturally sensitive pain care. *Pain Management Nursing, 1*(3 Suppl 1), 16–22. https://doi.org/10.1053/jpmn.2000.9761

Lyon, M. E., Jacobs, S., Briggs, L., Cheng, Y. I., & Wang, J. (2014). A longitudinal, randomized, controlled trial of advance care planning for teens with cancer: Anxiety, depression, quality of life, advance directives, spirituality. *Journal of Adolescent Health, 54*(6), 710–717. https://doi.org/10.1016/j.jadohealth.2013.10.206

Medicare.gov. (2023). *Skilled nursing facility (SNF) care*. https://www.medicare.gov/coverage/skilled-nursing-facility-snf-care

Napier, A. D., Ancarno, C., Butler, B., Calabrese, J., Chater, A., Chatterjee, H., Guesnet, F., Horne, R., Jacyna, S., Jadhav, S., Macdonald, A., Neuendorf, U., Parkhurst, A., Reynolds, R., Scambler, G., Shamdasani, S., Smith, S. Z., Stougaard-Nielsen, J., Thomson, L., ... Woolf, K. (2014). Culture and health. *The Lancet, 384*(9954), 1607–1639. https://doi.org/10.1016/S0140-6736(14)61603-2

National Association of Social Workers. (2004). *NASW standards for social work practice in palliative and end of life care*. NASW Press.

National Association of Social Workers. (2015). *Standards and indicators for cultural competence in social work practice*. NASW Press.

National Hospice and Palliative Care Organization. (2023). *NHPCO facts and figures: Hospice care in America*. https://allianceforcareathome.org/resource/2025-facts-and-figures-executive-summary/

Naylor, M. D., Bowles, K. H., McCauley, K. M., Maccoy, M. C., Maislin, G., Pauly, M. V., & Krakauer, R. (2013). High-value transitional care: Translation of research into practice. *Journal of Evaluation in Clinical Practice, 19*(5), 727–733. https://doi.org/10.1111/j.1365-2753.2011.01659.x

Neimeyer, R. A. (Ed.). (2001). *Meaning reconstruction and the experience of loss*. American Psychological Association.

Padela, A. I., & del Pozo, P. R. (2011). Muslim patients and cross-gender physical examinations. *Journal of General Internal Medicine, 26*(11), 1357. https://doi.org/10.1007/s11606-011-1797-8

Papadatou, D. (2009). *In the face of death: Professionals who care for the dying and the bereaved*. Springer Publishing Company.

Pettigrew, T. F., & Tropp, L. R. (2006). A meta-analytic test of intergroup contact theory. *Journal of Personality and Social Psychology, 90*(5), 751–783. https://doi.org/10.1037/0022-3514.90.5.751

Phelan, S. M., Burgess, D. J., Yeazel, M. W., Hellerstedt, W. L., Griffin, J. M., & van Ryn, M. (2015). Impact of weight bias and stigma on quality of care and outcomes for patients with obesity. *Obesity Reviews, 16*(4), 319–326. https://doi.org/10.1111/obr.12266

Prigerson, H. G., Horowitz, M. J., Jacobs, S. C., Parkes, C. M., Aslan, M., Goodkin, K., Raphael, B., Marwit, S. J., Wortman, C., Neimeyer, R. A., Bonanno, G., Block, S. D., Kissane, D., Boelen, P., Maercker, A., Litz, B. T., Johnson, J. G., First, M. B., & Maciejewski, P. K. (2009). Prolonged grief disorder: Psychometric validation of criteria proposed for DSM-V and ICD-11. *PLoS Medicine, 6*(8), e1000121. https://doi.org/10.1371/journal.pmed.1000121

Puchalski, C., Ferrell, B., Virani, R., Otis-Green, S., Baird, P., Bull, J., Chochinov, H., Handzo, G., Nelson-Becker, H., Prince-Paul, M., Pugliese, K., & Sulmasy, D. (2009). Improving the quality of spiritual care as a dimension of palliative care: The report of the Consensus Conference. *Journal of Palliative Medicine, 12*(10), 885–904. https://doi.org/10.1089/jpm.2009.0142

Rando, T. A. (2000). *Clinical dimensions of anticipatory mourning: Theory and practice in working with the dying, their loved ones, and their caregivers*. Research Press.

Rathert, C., Wyrwich, M. D., & Boren, S. A. (2013). Patient-centered care and outcomes: A systematic review of the literature. *Medical Care Research and Review, 70*(4), 351–379. https://doi.org/10.1177/1077558712465774

Reinhard, S. C., Given, B., Petlick, N. H., & Bemis, A. (2008). Supporting family caregivers in providing care. In R. G. Hughes (Ed.), *Patient safety and quality: An evidence-based handbook for nurses* (Chapter 14). Agency for Healthcare Research and Quality.

Roberts, A. R. (Ed.). (2005). *Crisis intervention handbook: Assessment, treatment, and research* (3rd ed.). Oxford University Press.

Roberts, A. R., & Everly, G. S. (2006). A meta-analysis of 36 crisis intervention studies. *Brief Treatment and Crisis Intervention, 6*(1), 10–21. https://doi.org/10.1093/brief-treatment/mhj006

Rosenblatt, P. C. (2008). Grief across cultures: A review and research agenda. In M. S. Stroebe, R. O. Hansson, H. Schut, & W. Stroebe (Eds.), *Handbook of bereavement research and practice: Advances in theory and intervention* (pp. 207–222). American Psychological Association.

Sabatino, C. P. (2010). The evolution of health care advance planning law and policy. *Milbank Quarterly, 88*(2), 211–239. https://doi.org/10.1111/j.1468-0009.2010.00596.x

Schicktanz, S., Raz, A., & Shalev, C. (2010). The cultural context of patient autonomy and doctor-patient relationship: Case studies from Israel and Germany. *Medicine, Health Care and Philosophy, 13*(3), 169–179. https://doi.org/10.1007/s11019-009-9230-9

Searight, H. R., & Gafford, J. (2005). Cultural diversity at the end of life: Issues and guidelines for family physicians. *American Family Physician, 71*(3), 515–522.

Shear, M. K. (2015). Complicated grief. *New England Journal of Medicine, 372*(2), 153–160. https://doi.org/10.1056/NEJMcp1315618

Shear, M. K., Reynolds, C. F., Simon, N. M., Zisook, S., Wang, Y., Mauro, C., Duan, N., Lebowitz, B., & Skritskaya, N. (2016). Optimizing treatment of complicated grief: A randomized clinical trial. *JAMA Psychiatry, 73*(7), 685–694. https://doi.org/10.1001/jamapsychiatry.2016.0892

Shepperd, S., Lannin, N. A., Clemson, L. M., McCluskey, A., Cameron, I. D., & Barras, S. L. (2013). Discharge planning from hospital to home. *Cochrane Database of Systematic Reviews, 1*, CD000313. https://doi.org/10.1002/14651858.CD000313.pub4

Sommers, B. D., & Singh, S. (2021). Association of pandemic-era changes in health insurance coverage with cardiovascular disease access and affordability. *JAMA Cardiology, 6*(12), 1429–1431. https://doi.org/10.1001/jamacardio.2021.3973

Stein, G. L., Beckerman, N. L., & Sherman, P. A. (2010). Lesbian and gay elders and long-term care: Identifying the unique psychosocial perspectives and challenges. *Journal of Gerontological Social Work, 53*(5), 421–435. https://doi.org/10.1080/01634372.2010.496478

Stroebe, M., & Schut, H. (1999). The dual process model of coping with bereavement: Rationale and description. *Death Studies, 23*(3), 197–224. https://doi.org/10.1080/074811899201046

Stroebe, M., & Schut, H. (2010). The dual process model of coping with bereavement: A decade on. *Omega, 61*(4), 273–289. https://doi.org/10.2190/OM.61.4.b

Sudore, R. L., & Fried, T. R. (2010). Redefining the "planning" in advance care planning: Preparing for end-of-life decision making. *Annals of Internal Medicine, 153*(4), 256–261. https://doi.org/10.7326/0003-4819-153-4-201008170-00008

Sudore, R. L., Lum, H. D., You, J. J., Hanson, L. C., Meier, D. E., Pantilat, S. Z., Matlock, D. D., Rietjens, J. A. C., Korfage, I. J., Ritchie, C. S., Kutner, J. S., Teno, J. M., Thomas, J., McMahan, R. D., & Heyland, D. K. (2017). Defining advance care planning for adults: A consensus definition from a multidisciplinary Delphi panel. *Journal of Pain and Symptom Management, 53*(5), 821–832. https://doi.org/10.1016/j.jpainsymman.2016.12.331

Tervalon, M., & Murray-García, J. (1998). Cultural humility versus cultural competence: A critical distinction in defining physician training outcomes in multicultural education. *Journal of Health Care for the Poor and Underserved, 9*(2), 117–125. https://doi.org/10.1353/hpu.2010.0233

U.S. Census Bureau. (2019). *Language spoken at home*. American Community Survey. https://data.census.gov

U.S. Department of Health and Human Services. (1991). *Patient Self-Determination Act of 1990*. Federal Register, *56*(22), 8508–8518.

U.S. Department of Health and Human Services. (2003). *Guidance to federal financial assistance recipients regarding Title VI prohibition against national origin discrimination affecting limited English proficient persons*. 68 Fed. Reg. 47311.

van Boekel, L. C., Brouwers, E. P., van Weeghel, J., & Garretsen, H. F. (2013). Stigma among health professionals towards patients with substance use disorders and its consequences for healthcare delivery: Systematic review. *Drug and Alcohol Dependence, 131*(1–2), 23–35. https://doi.org/10.1016/j.drugalcdep.2013.02.018

kindyn, M., & Burke, J. (2000). The effect of patient race and socio-economic status on physicians' perceptions of patients. *Social Science & Medicine, 50*(6), 813–828. https://doi.org/10.1016/S0277-9536(99)00338-X

Wallace, R., Hughes-Cromwick, P., Mull, H., & Khasnabis, S. (2005). Access to health care and nonemergency medical transportation: Two missing links. *Transportation Research Record, 1924*(1), 76–84. https://doi.org/10.1177/0361198105192400110

Worden, J. W. (2018). *Grief counseling and grief therapy: A handbook for the mental health practitioner* (5th ed.). Springer Publishing Company.

World Health Organization. (2008). *Closing the gap in a generation: Health equity through action on the social determinants of health*. WHO Commission on Social Determinants of Health.

Yadav, K. N., Gabler, N. B., Cooney, E., Kent, S., Kim, J., Herbst, N., Mante, A., Halpern, S. D., & Courtright, K. R. (2017). Approximately one in three US adults completes any type of advance directive for end-of-life care. *Health Affairs, 36*(7), 1244–1251. https://doi.org/10.1377/hlthaff.2017.0175

Yeager, K. A., & Bauer-Wu, S. (2013). Cultural humility: Essential foundation for clinical researchers. *Applied Nursing Research, 26*(4), 251–256. https://doi.org/10.1016/j.apnr.2013.06.008

Section III

# Ethics, Advocacy, and Equity

Medical social workers occupy a unique position within health care systems, serving simultaneously as members of institutional teams and as advocates for patient rights and social justice. This dual role creates both opportunities and tensions. While technical competence and relational skills prove essential, they remain insufficient without ethical clarity and commitment to advocacy.

This section addresses the ethical foundations and justice imperatives that distinguish social work from other health care professions. Social work's historical roots in social reform and its professional commitment to social justice position medical social workers as moral anchors within health care systems increasingly dominated by efficiency, cost containment, and biomedical priorities (Reamer, 2013). When institutional pressures conflict with patient needs, when vulnerable populations face discrimination, when systems perpetuate injustice, social workers must speak truth to power while maintaining professional relationships and institutional effectiveness.

The NASW Code of Ethics (2021) articulates core values including service, social justice, dignity and worth of the person, importance of human relationships, integrity, and competence. These values demand more than technical skill application; they require ongoing critical reflection about power, privilege, and professional responsibility. Medical social workers practice ethics daily through small decisions about whose voices are centered, which concerns receive attention, and how scarce resources are allocated.

The five chapters in this section strengthen ethical reasoning and advocacy capacity:

**Chapter 11: Protecting Patient Rights** examines autonomy, informed consent, and capacity assessment, exploring social work's role in safeguarding self-determination within systems that may prioritize efficiency or paternalism over patient choice.

**Chapter 12: Mandated Reporting in Health Care** addresses the legal and ethical complexities of mandatory reporting obligations, balancing protection of vulnerable individuals with respect for therapeutic relationships and patient autonomy.

**Chapter 13: Ethical Decision-Making in Complex Cases** provides frameworks for navigating moral dilemmas common in medical settings, including conflicts between principles, stakeholder disagreements, and situations where all available options create harm.

**Chapter 14: Health Equity and Social Justice** analyzes how social determinants of health and structural inequities shape health outcomes, positioning social workers as agents of both individual advocacy and systemic change.

**Chapter 15: Understanding Health Care Laws and Policies** explores key legal frameworks affecting practice including HIPAA, EMTALA, ADA, and mental health laws, examining how legal knowledge strengthens advocacy while identifying where laws themselves perpetuate injustice.

These chapters affirm that ethical practice extends beyond avoiding violations to proactively advancing justice, challenging oppression, and centering the voices of marginalized populations. Social workers serve not merely as system navigators helping individuals adapt to unjust structures but as change agents working to transform systems themselves.

CHAPTER 11

# Protecting Patient Rights

## Learning Objectives

By the end of this chapter, you will be able to do the following:

- Apply bioethical principles of autonomy, beneficence, non-maleficence, and justice to clinical situations
- Conduct systematic capacity assessments distinguishing capacity from competency
- Identify situations where informed consent processes are compromised
- Advocate for shared decision-making and patient-centered care
- Navigate conflicts between patient autonomy and family preferences or clinical recommendations

## Bioethical Foundations of Patient Rights

Modern biomedical ethics emerged partly in response to historical abuses including Nazi medical experiments, the Tuskegee Syphilis Study, and routine paternalism in physician-patient relationships that denied patients information and choice (Jonsen, 2000). The Belmont Report (1979) established three foundational principles for research ethics that subsequently influenced clinical ethics: respect for persons (honoring autonomy), beneficence (maximizing benefits), and justice (fair distribution of burdens and benefits). Beauchamp and Childress (2019) expanded this framework adding non-maleficence (avoiding harm), creating the four principles most commonly invoked in health care ethics.

**Autonomy** prioritizes individual self-determination, the right to make decisions about one's own body and medical treatment based on personal values, beliefs, and preferences. Respecting autonomy requires providing adequate information, ensuring understanding, and honoring choices even when practitioners disagree. Autonomy is not absolute; limitations exist when choices directly harm others or when individuals lack decision-making capacity. However, contemporary bioethics presumes competent adults possess autonomy unless evidence suggests otherwise (Beauchamp & Childress, 2019).

**Beneficence** obligates health care professionals to act in patients' best interests, promoting well-being and preventing or removing harm. Historically, beneficence dominated medical ethics, with physicians making paternalistic decisions they deemed beneficial without significant patient input. Contemporary bioethics maintains beneficence as important but subordinate to autonomy when both cannot be simultaneously honored.

**Non-maleficence**, the obligation to "first, do no harm," requires that interventions not inflict suffering, injury, or death unnecessarily. This principle proves particularly relevant in end-of-life decisions where aggressive treatment may prolong life while creating significant suffering. Balancing life prolongation against quality of life requires nuanced ethical reasoning and patient value clarification.

**Justice** demands fair, equitable, and appropriate treatment, including fair resource allocation and freedom from discrimination. Justice operates at both micro levels (individual patient interactions) and macro levels (system policies and resource distribution). Social workers' commitment to social justice extends traditional bioethics' focus on individual cases to include structural inequities affecting health and health care access.

Medical social workers apply these principles daily, often navigating conflicts between them. When a patient refuses recommended treatment (autonomy) that would likely benefit them (beneficence), which principle takes precedence? When family members request aggressive treatment for a dying patient whose suffering would increase (non-maleficence), how should practitioners respond? When limited resources cannot serve all who need them (justice), how are allocation decisions made? These questions lack simple answers but require systematic ethical reasoning.

## Informed Consent: More Than a Signature

Informed consent represents autonomy in practice, the process ensuring patients understand their medical situations sufficiently to make voluntary, informed decisions. True informed consent requires satisfaction of multiple conditions (Faden & Beauchamp, 1986):

**Adequate information disclosure** includes diagnosis, prognosis, proposed treatment with expected benefits and risks, alternative treatments with their benefits and risks, and consequences of declining treatment. Information must be provided in language appropriate to the patient's health literacy, cultural background, and language, avoiding medical jargon that obscures rather than clarifies.

**Comprehension** extends beyond information provision to ensuring understanding. Practitioners must verify that patients grasp information provided, its implications for them personally, and the choices they face. The teach-back method addresses comprehension: "Can you explain in your own words what we discussed?" or "What will you tell your family about the treatment options?" Patients with cognitive impairments, low health literacy, limited English proficiency, or high anxiety may receive information but fail to comprehend it adequately.

**Voluntariness** requires freedom from coercion, manipulation, or undue influence. Subtle pressures compromise voluntariness: time pressure to decide quickly, framing options to favor particular choices, emotional manipulation through fear or guilt, or family pressure overriding patient preferences. Hospitalized patients experience inherent vulnerability; social workers protect voluntariness by ensuring patients understand they can refuse treatment, ask questions, request time to consider options, and consult others before deciding (Beauchamp & Childress, 2019).

**Decision-making capacity** represents the cognitive and emotional ability to make informed health decisions. Capacity assessment addresses whether patients can understand relevant information, appreciate how information applies to their situation, reason through options and consequences, and communicate a choice. Capacity exists along a continuum rather than as absolute presence or absence, varies across decisions of different complexity, and may fluctuate over time with mental status changes (Appelbaum, 2007).

Common informed consent violations include obtaining signatures without adequate explanation, providing information so technical that comprehension is impossible, pressuring patients toward particular choices through framing or urgency, obtaining consent from family members when patients retain capacity, and proceeding with treatment when patients clearly lack comprehension despite receiving information. Social workers intervene when observing compromised consent processes, advocating for clearer communication, additional time, professional interpretation, or capacity evaluation.

## Assessing Decision-Making Capacity

Capacity assessment represents a crucial social work function, particularly given social workers' expertise in psychosocial functioning and cognitive assessment. While physicians may request capacity evaluations, social workers, psychologists, and psychiatrists all contribute. Understanding capacity assessment principles enables effective participation in this process (Appelbaum, 2007).

**Capacity Versus Competency:** Capacity represents a clinical determination made by health care professionals regarding functional ability to make specific health decisions. Competency represents a legal status determined by courts through formal proceedings. Competent adults are presumed to possess capacity unless evidence suggests otherwise. A patient may be legally competent (no court has declared them incompetent) while lacking capacity for complex health decisions due to delirium, dementia, or severe mental illness. Conversely, individuals under guardianship (legally incompetent) may retain capacity for certain decisions depending on guardianship scope.

**Capacity Standards:** Various standards for capacity exist, with selection depending on decision significance and risk. The sliding scale approach applies more stringent standards to decisions carrying greater risk or irreversibility. Expressing a choice, the lowest standard, simply requires communicating a preference. Understanding relevant information requires grasping diagnosis, treatment options, and their implications. Appreciation of the situation demands recognizing how information applies personally, not just abstract comprehension. Rational manipulation of information involves comparing options based on personal values and logical reasoning. Most clinicians apply standards requiring understanding, appreciation, and reasoning for significant medical decisions (Grisso & Appelbaum, 1998).

**The capacity assessment process** involves

1. **Clarifying the specific decision** requiring capacity assessment (global capacity determinations are inappropriate; capacity is decision-specific)
2. **Gathering background information** about cognitive function, psychiatric symptoms, medications affecting cognition, and previous capacity determinations
3. **Explaining the medical situation** in clear language and assessing understanding through open-ended questions
4. **Exploring appreciation** by asking how the information applies to the patient personally
5. **Examining reasoning** by asking patients to compare options and explain their rationale
6. **Considering fluctuating capacity** and whether temporary impairments might resolve with treatment
7. **Documenting findings** clearly, specifying what decision is addressed, what standards were applied, and the basis for conclusions

**Red flags suggesting impaired capacity:** Inability to state diagnosis or reason for hospitalization, inability to name treatment options despite repeated explanation, belief that illness is not real or that they are not sick (lack of insight), inability to weigh risks and benefits of options, choices clearly inconsistent with previously stated values without explanation, delusional thinking directly relevant to the decision, severe depression creating hopelessness and passive acceptance, and disorganized thinking preventing logical reasoning. However, these suggest rather than prove incapacity; systematic assessment remains necessary.

**When capacity is lacking:** If patients lack capacity, surrogate decision-makers assume responsibility. The hierarchy typically follows health care agent designated through medical power of attorney, court-appointed guardian, spouse, adult children, parents, siblings, then other relatives. Surrogates should make substituted judgments based on what the patient would want if able to decide, determined from previous statements, values, and life choices. When patient preferences cannot be determined, surrogates make best interest decisions focused on maximizing benefit and minimizing harm. Social workers support surrogates by explaining the decision, clarifying the patient's known values, facilitating family consensus when possible, and providing emotional support during difficult choices (Rid & Wendler, 2010).

## Protecting Autonomy in Vulnerable Populations

Certain patient populations face heightened autonomy risks, requiring particular social work vigilance.

**Patients with cognitive impairment:** Dementia, delirium, intellectual disabilities, and traumatic brain injury affect but do not necessarily eliminate capacity. Practitioners should maximize capacity through optimal timing (morning, when less confused), environmental modifications (quiet, familiar spaces), communication adaptations (simple language, visual aids), and treating reversible causes of impairment (infection, medications, metabolic disturbances). Dismissing cognitively impaired patients as incapable without thorough assessment violates autonomy (Moye et al., 2013).

**Psychiatric patients:** Mental illness does not equal incapacity. Depression, anxiety, schizophrenia, and bipolar disorder may or may not impair decision-making capacity depending on symptom severity and relevance to the specific decision. Psychotic patients may retain capacity for many decisions if delusions do not affect judgment about the matter at hand. Refusal of psychiatric treatment demands careful capacity assessment given the dilemma that the condition being refused treatment for may impair capacity to refuse. Social workers advocate against reflexive capacity dismissal while recognizing that severe psychiatric symptoms sometimes genuinely impair decision-making (Srebnik & La Fond, 1999).

**Non-English-speaking patients:** Language barriers dramatically compromise informed consent. When professional interpretation is unavailable or inadequate, patients cannot provide informed consent because information exchange proves impossible. Using family members as interpreters creates additional problems: information filtering, role confusion, and privacy violations. Social workers must advocate vigorously for professional interpretation, recognizing that proceeding without it violates both autonomy and standard of care (Karliner et al., 2007).

**Elderly patients:** Ageism leads to autonomy violations when families or providers dismiss elder preferences as confused, stubborn, or incompetent without actual capacity evaluation. Older adults retain autonomy even when making choices that family members or providers consider unwise. Risk-averse choices limiting independence may reflect realistic assessment of limitations rather than impaired judgment. Social workers challenge ageist assumptions while conducting genuine capacity assessments when concerns arise.

**Patients experiencing homelessness:** This population faces unique autonomy challenges. Leaving "against medical advice" from the hospital may be labeled noncompliant when actually representing rational choice given lack of safe housing. Treatment refusal may reflect past medical trauma or distrust rather than incapacity. Social workers consider how structural barriers and past experiences shape apparently "poor" decisions before concluding capacity is absent.

## Shared Decision-Making as Autonomy in Practice

Shared decision-making (SDM) operationalizes respect for autonomy through collaborative processes where clinicians and patients jointly make treatment decisions based on both medical evidence and patient values (Charles et al., 1997). Unlike paternalistic models where physicians decide or informed choice models where physicians present information and patients decide alone, SDM recognizes that optimal decisions require integrating clinical expertise with patient knowledge of their own values, goals, and life circumstances.

**Core Elements of Shared Decision-Making:**

1. **Both parties acknowledge that decisions require making** and collaboration would be beneficial
2. **Clinicians present options** including benefits, harms, and uncertainties in accessible language

3. **Patients are supported** to explore values, preferences, and concerns through deliberative discussion
4. **Decision-making responsibility is shared** with neither party dominating
5. **Agreement is reached** about treatment plan going forward

Research demonstrates SDM benefits including increased patient satisfaction, improved adherence, reduced decisional conflict and regret, and in some cases better health outcomes (Stiggelbout et al., 2015). SDM proves particularly valuable for preference-sensitive decisions where multiple reasonable options exist without clear medical superiority, where decisions involve values trade-offs, or where consequences include quality of life impacts.

**Social work roles in promoting SDM:** Social workers facilitate SDM by clarifying patient values and goals through motivational interviewing techniques, translating medical information into understandable language, identifying barriers to shared processes including power differentials or cultural expectations, advocating with medical teams for patient inclusion in decisions, and documenting patient preferences and values to inform future decisions. SDM represents autonomy respect through relationship rather than through isolated consent signatures.

## Conflicts Between Autonomy and Other Values

Autonomy regularly conflicts with other ethical principles or practical considerations, requiring deliberate ethical reasoning.

**Autonomy versus beneficence:** When patients refuse treatments clinicians believe would substantially benefit them, conflict emerges between respecting autonomy and promoting wellbeing. Competent adult patients have legal and ethical rights to refuse treatment, including life-saving treatment, even when refusal appears irrational to observers. Social workers may feel distress when patients make choices that will likely cause harm, creating moral distress when professional obligations conflict with personal values. Response strategies include verifying capacity, ensuring decisions are truly informed and voluntary, exploring reasons for refusal which may reveal modifiable concerns, and accepting that honoring autonomy sometimes means witnessing choices we would not make (Brock, 2008).

**Individual autonomy versus family values:** Some cultures and families prioritize collective decision-making over individual autonomy, viewing autonomous choice as selfish individualism rather than valued independence. Families may request that patients not be told terminal prognoses or may wish to make treatment decisions for incapacitated relatives in ways inconsistent with patient's previously stated preferences. Social workers navigate these tensions by exploring with patients their own preferences for decision-making involvement, honoring diverse cultural practices while protecting patient voice, facilitating family meetings to build understanding, and recognizing that protecting autonomy sometimes means supporting family-centered decision-making when that is the patient's autonomous preference (Johnstone & Kanitsaki, 2009).

**Autonomy versus limited resources:** When resources are scarce (ICU beds, transplant organs, expensive medications), honoring every patient's autonomous choice becomes impossible. Justice demands fair allocation, potentially overriding some individual preferences. Social workers participate in these ethically fraught decisions by advocating for transparent, equitable allocation processes; ensuring that vulnerable populations are not systematically disadvantaged; and supporting patients who do not receive preferred resources through grief processes and alternative planning.

## Critical Thinking Questions

1. Analyze informed consent through a critical theory lens examining power relations inherent in medical encounters. How do structural factors including race, class, gender, and disability status

affect whose autonomy is respected versus questioned? What changes to consent processes would address these power imbalances?

2. Evaluate the concept of decision-making capacity as socially constructed. How do cultural values about rational thinking, emotional expression, and family involvement shape what assessors interpret as capacity versus incapacity? What alternative frameworks might honor diverse forms of sound decision-making?
3. Critique the bioethical principle of autonomy from communitarian or care ethics perspectives. How might emphasizing individual autonomy harm individuals who define themselves through relationships and communities? What ethical frameworks better honor interdependence while protecting against coercion?
4. Examine the concept of "rational" decision-making underlying capacity assessment. How do emotion, intuition, spirituality, and other non-rational factors appropriately influence health decisions? When does labeling emotional decisions as irrational reflect professional bias rather than genuine incapacity?

## Key Takeaways

- Four principles (autonomy, beneficence, non-maleficence, justice) provide foundational framework for biomedical ethics, though they often conflict requiring careful reasoning.
- Informed consent requires more than signatures; true consent demands adequate information disclosure, patient comprehension, voluntariness, and decision-making capacity.
- Capacity assessment is decision-specific, exists on a continuum, and requires systematic evaluation of understanding, appreciation, reasoning, and choice expression.
- Vulnerable populations including those with cognitive impairment, psychiatric illness, language barriers, and marginalized identities face heightened autonomy risks requiring advocacy.
- Shared decision-making operationalizes autonomy through collaborative processes integrating clinical evidence with patient values and preferences.
- Conflicts between autonomy and other ethical principles or practical constraints require deliberate ethical reasoning rather than automatic autonomy prioritization.

CHAPTER 12

# Mandated Reporting in Healthcare

## Learning Objectives

By the end of this chapter, you will be able to do the following:

- Identify situations requiring mandated reporting under state and federal laws
- Navigate the legal and ethical complexities of reporting obligations
- Balance protection of vulnerable individuals with therapeutic relationships and patient autonomy
- Complete mandated reports accurately and thoroughly
- Address the emotional and relational impacts of mandatory reporting

## Legal Foundations of Mandated Reporting

Mandated reporting laws require designated professionals including social workers to report suspected abuse, neglect, or exploitation of vulnerable populations to appropriate authorities. These laws emerged from recognition that vulnerable individuals (children, elders, people with disabilities) may be unable to report abuse themselves and that early intervention can prevent escalating harm (Mathews & Bross, 2008). All 50 states have child abuse reporting laws; elder abuse reporting laws exist in most jurisdictions with variations in who must report and what conditions trigger reporting.

**Mandatory reporters** typically include health care professionals (physicians, nurses, social workers), educators, childcare providers, law enforcement, and mental health professionals. The specific list varies by state. Some states designate all citizens as mandated reporters (universal reporting), while others specify professions. Social workers are mandated reporters in all jurisdictions where such laws exist, meaning failure to report when legally obligated constitutes a criminal misdemeanor, professional ethics violation, and potential civil liability (Kalichman, 1999).

**Reasonable suspicion standard:** Mandated reporters must report when they have reasonable suspicion or reasonable cause to believe that abuse, neglect, or exploitation has occurred or is occurring. Reasonable suspicion requires more than speculation but less than proof or certainty. Reporters need not investigate or determine conclusively that abuse occurred; that investigation role belongs to child protective services (CPS), adult protective services (APS), or law enforcement. The low threshold aims to prevent underreporting and enable investigation by specialized authorities (Levi & Portwood, 2011).

Indicators creating reasonable suspicion vary but may include unexplained injuries inconsistent with provided explanations, a pattern of injuries suggesting abuse rather than accidents, severe neglect evidenced by malnutrition or poor hygiene, patient statements suggesting abuse or fear, caregiver behavior suggesting controlling or abusive dynamics, a withholding of necessary medical care, or signs of financial exploitation. Social workers develop pattern recognition over time; suspicious presentations warrant reporting even when individual indicators might have innocent explanations.

**Immunity provisions:** All mandated reporting statutes provide immunity from civil and criminal liability for reporters who make reports in good faith, even if investigation determines abuse did not occur. This immunity encourages reporting by protecting well-intentioned professionals from lawsuits by accused individuals. However, immunity does not extend to reckless or malicious false reports. Bad faith reporting or using reporting as weapon in custody disputes constitutes abuse of reporting systems and may result in liability (Alvarez et al., 2004).

**Reporting procedures:** Each state maintains child abuse hotlines and elder/adult abuse reporting systems with specific procedures. Generally, reporting involves making an immediate verbal report (phone call) followed by written report within specified timeframes (typically 24-72 hours). Reports must include available information about the victim, the abuse or neglect suspected, the basis for suspicion, the reporter's identity and contact information, and any relevant history. Some jurisdictions accept anonymous reports, though mandated reporters should identify themselves, given their legal obligations. Social workers should document in clinical records that reports were made, including dates, times, recipient agencies, and report contents.

## Child Abuse and Neglect Reporting

Child abuse and neglect reporting represents the most established and comprehensive mandated reporting system. Federal law (Child Abuse Prevention and Treatment Act) provides framework and funding, while state laws define specific reportable conditions and procedures (Administration for Children and Families, 2019).

### Reportable Conditions

While definitions vary by state, generally, reportable child abuse and neglect include the following.

1. **Physical abuse:** Non-accidental physical injury including striking, burning, biting, shaking, or otherwise physically harming children. Indicators include bruises in various healing stages, injuries to non-accessible areas (inner thighs, back, buttocks), patterned injuries (belt marks, grab marks), burns with clear boundaries suggesting immersion or contact with hot objects, and explanations inconsistent with injury patterns or developmental capabilities.
2. **Sexual abuse:** Any sexual contact with a child, exposure to sexual material or activities, or exploitation including child pornography. Indicators may include age-inappropriate sexual knowledge or behavior, genital injuries or infections, regression in previously mastered skills, nightmares, fear of particular individuals, and disclosures. Child sexual abuse victims often delay disclosure or recant due to fear, loyalty, or coercion, making initial disclosures particularly important.
3. **Emotional/psychological abuse:** Patterns of behavior causing emotional harm including excessive criticism, threats, rejection, isolation, or witnessing domestic violence. This proves hardest to identify and substantiate but creates significant developmental harm.
4. **Neglect:** Failure to provide basic needs including food, shelter, medical care, supervision, or education. Medical neglect occurs when caregivers refuse or fail to obtain necessary medical treatment for serious conditions. Chronic inadequate supervision leaving young children alone or with inappropriate caregivers constitutes neglect.
5. **Special considerations in medical settings:** Hospitals encounter potential child abuse regularly given that abused children often present for medical care. Unexplained injuries, delayed care-seeking for serious injuries, inconsistent explanations from caregivers, and a pattern of repeated injuries that raises questions all warrant reporting. Medical social workers collaborate with child

abuse pediatricians and hospital abuse teams when these exist, but individual reporting obligations remain even when teams are involved. Differential diagnosis must consider non-abusive causes (bleeding disorders, bone fragility conditions, cultural practices like cupping or coining) while maintaining low reporting threshold given reasonable suspicion standard (Flaherty et al., 2014).

# Elder Abuse and Vulnerable Adult Reporting

Elder abuse affects approximately 10% of older adults annually, with rates likely higher due to significant underreporting (Acierno et al., 2010). Unlike child abuse systems with universal CPS agencies, elder abuse response systems vary substantially across states. Some states have robust APS agencies with investigative authority; others have minimal systems relying primarily on law enforcement.

## Types of Elder/Vulnerable Adult Abuse

1. **Physical abuse:** Inflicting physical pain or injury through hitting, pushing, slapping, burning, restraining, or force-feeding. Physical abuse may be perpetrated by family caregivers, paid caregivers, or facility staff.
2. **Emotional/psychological abuse:** Verbal assaults, threats, intimidation, humiliation, or isolation causing emotional distress. This includes treating elders like children, ignoring them, or systematically excluding them from decisions.
3. **Sexual abuse:** Any nonconsensual sexual contact with older adults or adults with disabilities who cannot consent due to cognitive impairment. Sexual abuse in nursing homes and by caregivers occurs more frequently than commonly recognized.
4. **Financial exploitation:** Illegal or improper use of an elder's funds, property, or assets through theft, fraud, or undue influence. This includes family members or caregivers taking money, coercing changes to wills or financial documents, or using power of attorney inappropriately. Financial exploitation often co-occurs with other abuse forms, as perpetrators isolate victims to prevent detection.
5. **Neglect:** Failure to provide necessary care including food, water, medication, medical care, hygiene assistance, or safe living conditions. Neglect may be intentional or result from caregiver inability to provide adequate care due to their own impairments, lack of knowledge, or resource limitations. Self-neglect, where individuals fail to care for themselves, is reportable in some states though it raises complex autonomy questions.

## Indicators of Elder Abuse

Unexplained injuries, pressure ulcers suggesting inadequate care, malnutrition or dehydration without medical explanation, poor hygiene despite caregiver presence, oversedation or under-medication, fear of particular individuals, reluctance to speak in caregiver's presence, signs of restraint use, and sudden changes in financial circumstances warrant exploration. Social workers should interview elders privately when possible, as abused individuals may be unable to speak freely with abusers present. However, cognitive impairment may prevent reliable reporting, necessitating reliance on suspicious patterns.

## Autonomy Tensions

Elder abuse reporting creates unique autonomy tensions absent in child abuse cases. Competent older adults have the right to refuse interventions even when being abused, to remain in unsafe situations if they choose, and to decline prosecution of abusers. APS cannot remove competent adults from dangerous situations against their will the way that CPS can remove endangered children. This creates frustration when social workers identify abuse but victims refuse to leave or press charges. Respecting autonomy means accepting that competent adults may make choices others view as dangerous, including remaining with abusive partners or family members. Social workers provide education about options, facilitate safety planning, maintain ongoing contact, and ensure that refusal of help represents informed choice rather than coercion or lack of understanding about alternatives (Nerenberg, 2008).

## Reporting Domestic Violence and Human Trafficking

### Domestic Violence

Mandated reporting requirements for domestic violence vary dramatically by state. Some states require reporting of all domestic violence injuries, others require reporting only when specific weapons are used or when injuries meet certain severity thresholds, and many states have no mandatory domestic violence reporting for competent adults. Social workers must know their state's specific requirements.

The mandatory domestic violence reporting debate reflects tensions between protection and autonomy. Proponents argue that mandatory reporting connects victims to resources, creates official records useful for protective orders and custody cases, and communicates societal intolerance of domestic violence. Opponents counter that mandatory reporting removes victim control, may escalate violence when victims are not ready to leave, discourages help-seeking if victims know disclosure means automatic reporting, and violates autonomy of competent adults who should decide whether to involve authorities (Rodriguez et al., 2001).

Research suggests mandatory reporting laws may have mixed effects. Some victims report feeling helped by mandatory reporting that motivated them to seek protection. Others report negative consequences including retaliatory violence, economic instability from partner arrest, and reluctance to seek health care due to reporting fears. Best practice in jurisdictions without mandatory reporting involves discussing safety, providing resources, supporting victims' choices, and respecting that leaving abusive relationships involves complex personal calculations about safety, economics, and children (Rodriguez et al., 2001).

### Human Trafficking

Federal law and increasing state laws require reporting of suspected human trafficking, including sex trafficking and labor trafficking. Health care settings encounter trafficking victims who present for medical care, often for injuries, reproductive health needs, or substance use treatment (Egyud et al., 2017). Indicators include signs of physical abuse, fearfulness or hypervigilance, individual unable to speak for themselves with controlling companion present, inconsistent explanation of injuries or living situation, and identifying marks suggesting trafficking (branding, tattoos). However, many trafficking victims will not disclose due to fear, trauma bonding, language barriers, or not self-identifying as victims. Social workers should screen sensitively, provide resources even without confirmation, and make reports when reasonable suspicion exists while recognizing that victim cooperation with investigation cannot be guaranteed.

## Ethical Complexities and Dilemmas in Mandated Reporting

While mandated reporting serves child and vulnerable adult protection, it creates genuine ethical tensions that social workers must navigate thoughtfully.

**Therapeutic relationship impact:** Mandated reporting can damage therapeutic relationships when patients experience reports as betrayal or violation of confidentiality. This proves particularly problematic in mental health and substance use treatment where therapeutic alliance is essential. Clients may disengage from needed services after reports, creating harm even when reporting was legally required. Social workers mitigate these impacts by discussing reporting obligations during informed consent, explaining reporting when it must occur, and maintaining empathy even as they fulfill legal duties (Weinstein et al., 2000).

**Cultural competence and reporting:** Cultural practices that appear as abuse or neglect within mainstream frameworks may represent accepted practices within particular communities. Coining, cupping, and other traditional healing practices can leave marks suggesting physical abuse. Co-sleeping arrangements may be reported as inadequate supervision despite being culturally normative and not actually dangerous. Extended family care common in some cultures may be seen as inadequate when official guardianship is absent. Social workers must distinguish genuine harm from cultural differences, avoiding both excessive reporting that disrupts families based on cultural misunderstanding and underreporting that leaves children at risk due to cultural relativism taken too far (Fontes, 2005).

**Self-determination conflicts:** Reporting decisions for competent adults with disabilities or elders who refuse intervention conflicts with self-determination principles. Social workers are ethically committed to client autonomy yet legally required to report suspected abuse. This creates moral distress when honoring legal obligations undermines ethical commitments. Careful capacity assessment becomes crucial; if individuals lack capacity due to cognitive impairment or undue influence, reporting serves protection. If individuals retain capacity and make informed choices to remain in risky situations, social workers must balance legal reporting obligations with respect for difficult autonomous choices.

**Uncertainty in reporting decisions:** The reasonable suspicion standard requires reporting even with significant uncertainty, yet reporting initiates investigations that may traumatize families, particularly in marginalized communities that have experienced systemic harm from child welfare systems. Underreporting endangers children and vulnerable adults; overreporting harms families and overwhelms protective services with unfounded cases. No perfect balance exists. Social workers should consult with supervisors and colleagues when uncertain, document reasoning, and err toward reporting when genuine safety concerns exist given immunity provisions and investigative agency authority to determine whether abuse occurred (Alvarez et al., 2004).

# Best Practices in Mandated Reporting

**Know state-specific requirements:** Reporting laws vary significantly. Social workers must thoroughly understand reporting obligations in states where they practice, including who must report, what conditions trigger reporting, to whom reports are made, and required timeframes. Professional organizations, state social work boards, and agencies' legal counsel provide authoritative guidance.

**Document thoroughly:** Clinical documentation should capture observations, statements, and reasoning supporting reporting decisions. Note indicators observed, statements by patients or others, patterns of concern, and basis for reasonable suspicion. If choosing not to report, document why suspicion did not rise to reasonable level including alternate explanations considered. Documentation provides legal protection and case continuity.

**Discuss reporting obligations during informed consent:** Transparency about confidentiality limits including mandated reporting builds trust and enables clients to make informed choices about what to disclose. Explain reporting obligations clearly: "I want you to know that most of what we discuss is confidential, but I am legally required to report if I suspect child abuse, elder abuse, or immediate danger to yourself or others."

**Maintain compassion when reporting:** Reporting need not be punitive or conveyed with judgment. Use empathetic language emphasizing concern and protection: "I care about your safety, and based on what you've shared, I'm required to make a report to adult protective services so they can help ensure you're safe." Maintain the therapeutic relationship post-report when possible, recognizing that reporting represents professional obligation rather than personal rejection.

**Collaborate with multidisciplinary teams:** When working in hospitals or agencies with abuse response teams, child abuse pediatricians, or forensic specialists, collaborate while recognizing that individual reporting obligations remain. Team consultation strengthens clinical decision-making but does not replace personal responsibility to report.

**Provide resources and follow-up:** Reporting to authorities represents one component of comprehensive response. Connect patients to domestic violence advocates, victim assistance services, legal aid, counseling, and other supports. Follow up after reports to assess patient safety and service connection.

**Seek consultation and supervision:** Mandated reporting decisions sometimes create uncertainty and emotional distress. Consult supervisors, colleagues, ethics committees, or legal counsel when appropriate. Debriefing after difficult reporting situations addresses vicarious trauma and supports ongoing ethical practice.

## Critical Thinking Questions

1. Analyze mandated reporting laws through a critical race theory lens. How do these laws disproportionately impact families of color and low-income families? What evidence exists regarding racial disparities in reporting, investigation, and substantiation? What reforms might address these inequities while maintaining child and vulnerable adult protection?
2. Evaluate the tension between mandated reporting and therapeutic alliance in mental health and substance use treatment. What does research reveal about reporting's impact on treatment engagement and outcomes? How might harm reduction principles inform reporting policy reform?
3. Critique the reasonable suspicion standard from an epistemological perspective. How do cultural background, implicit bias, and professional socialization shape what practitioners perceive as "reasonable" suspicion? What safeguards might reduce biased reporting while maintaining child and elder protection?
4. Examine the concept of mandated reporting for competent adults experiencing domestic violence through feminist ethics and autonomy frameworks. How do paternalism, victimization narratives, and state intervention interact in ways that may disempower rather than protect? What alternative approaches might better honor agency while addressing violence?

## Key Takeaways

- Mandated reporting laws require designated professionals including social workers to report suspected abuse, neglect, or exploitation of vulnerable populations based on reasonable suspicion standard.
- Reportable conditions include child physical abuse, sexual abuse, emotional abuse, and neglect; elder/vulnerable adult physical abuse, emotional abuse, sexual abuse, financial exploitation, and neglect; and in some jurisdictions, domestic violence and human trafficking.
- Reasonable suspicion requires more than speculation but less than certainty; immunity provisions protect good faith reporters from liability.
- Ethical tensions emerge between therapeutic relationships and reporting obligations, cultural practices and mainstream definitions of abuse, and protection versus autonomy for competent adults.
- Best practices include knowing state-specific requirements, transparent informed consent about reporting obligations, thorough documentation, compassionate communication, and consultation when uncertain.
- Mandated reporting serves protection but creates genuine ethical dilemmas requiring thoughtful navigation rather than automatic application.

CHAPTER 13

# Ethical Decision-Making in Complex Cases

## Learning Objectives

By the end of this chapter, you will be able to do the following:

- Apply systematic ethical decision-making frameworks to complex clinical situations
- Analyze ethical dilemmas using multiple theoretical perspectives
- Navigate conflicts between ethical principles, professional values, and institutional demands
- Recognize and address moral distress in health care practice
- Utilize ethics consultation and institutional resources appropriately

## The Nature of Ethical Dilemmas in Health Care

Ethical dilemmas arise when competing values, principles, or obligations create situations where any course of action involves compromise of important ethical commitments. Unlike technical problems with correct solutions, ethical dilemmas involve choosing between imperfect options, each carrying moral weight and potential harm (Beauchamp & Childress, 2019). Medical social workers regularly encounter ethical complexity including conflicts between patient autonomy and family wishes, beneficence and non-maleficence when interventions carry significant risks, individual patient needs and fair resource allocation, professional values and institutional policies, and legal obligations and ethical commitments.

**Common dilemmas:** Should life-sustaining treatment be continued when the patient previously stated preferences against aggressive care but family insists on everything possible? How should scarce resources be allocated when multiple patients have legitimate needs but insufficient services exist for all? What should be done when a patient lacks capacity and has no clear surrogate, requiring decisions about serious medical interventions? How should social workers respond when institutional policies conflict with patient needs or professional ethics? When does protection of vulnerable individuals justify overriding autonomy?

These dilemmas lack clear right answers discoverable through technical expertise. They require moral reasoning that balances principles, considers stakeholder perspectives, evaluates consequences, and remains consistent with professional values. Ethical decision-making frameworks provide systematic approaches to this complex reasoning, though they cannot eliminate the difficulty or guarantee consensus (Dolgoff et al., 2012).

## Theoretical Frameworks for Ethical Analysis

Multiple ethical theories provide lenses for analyzing dilemmas, each emphasizing different dimensions and reaching different conclusions. Understanding various frameworks strengthens ethical reasoning by revealing assumptions and expanding consideration of relevant factors.

**Principlism** applies the four principles discussed in Chapter 11 (autonomy, beneficence, non-maleficence, justice) to specific situations. When principles conflict, practitioners weigh which should take precedence given the context. Principlism's strength lies in its broad acceptance in health care and provision of common language for ethical discussion. Critics argue it provides insufficient guidance when principles conflict and lacks attention to relationships, emotions, and context (Beauchamp & Childress, 2019).

**Deontology** (duty-based ethics) emphasizes moral rules and duties regardless of consequences. Kantian deontology holds that some actions are inherently right or wrong based on whether they respect human dignity and treat people as ends rather than means. For example, lying is wrong even when lies might produce good outcomes because lying treats people as mere means to achieve one's goals. Deontology's strength involves clarity about duties and protection of individuals from being sacrificed for collective benefit. Limitations include potential rigidity and difficulty managing conflicting duties (Feldman, 1978).

**Utilitarianism** (consequentialism) judges actions by their consequences, deeming right those that maximize overall good (happiness, wellbeing, preference satisfaction) for the greatest number. Resource allocation decisions often invoke utilitarian reasoning: scarce organs should go to recipients with best outcomes, limited treatment should serve patients with greatest chance of benefit. Strengths include attention to actual outcomes and provision of framework for difficult allocation decisions. Critics note that utilitarianism may justify harming individuals for collective benefit, struggles with predicting consequences, and inadequately protects minority rights (Singer, 2011).

**Virtue ethics** focuses on character and what virtuous people would do rather than rules or consequences. Relevant virtues include compassion, courage, honesty, humility, and practical wisdom. Social workers exemplifying professional virtues make good decisions through cultivated character rather than rule application. Virtue ethics emphasizes moral development, relationship, and context but provides limited action guidance in specific dilemmas (Pellegrino & Thomasma, 1993).

**Care ethics** emerged from feminist scholarship challenging traditional ethics' emphasis on autonomy, rights, and justice while neglecting care, relationships, and interdependence. Care ethics emphasizes relationships, context, emotional engagement, and responsibility to vulnerable others. This framework aligns with social work's emphasis on relationships and attention to marginalized voices. Care ethics strengthens understanding of relational obligations but has been criticized for potentially reinforcing oppressive caregiver roles and providing insufficient guidance about conflicting care responsibilities (Held, 2006).

**Social justice framework** extends individual ethics to structural and systemic dimensions, examining how power, oppression, and inequity shape situations and solutions. This perspective asks who benefits from current arrangements, whose voices are excluded, and how interventions might reinforce or challenge unjust systems. Social justice ethics aligns with social work's professional commitment but creates tensions when individual and collective welfare conflict (Banerjee, 2011).

## The NASW Code of Ethics as Decision-Making Guide

The NASW Code of Ethics (2021) provides profession-specific ethical guidance organized around core values and principles. While the Code cannot resolve every dilemma, it establishes priorities and commitments guiding social work practice.

**Six Core Values:**

1. **Service** – Social workers' primary goal is helping people and addressing social problems
2. **Social Justice** – Social workers challenge social injustice and pursue change on behalf of vulnerable and oppressed populations
3. **Dignity and Worth of the Person** – Social workers respect the inherent dignity and worth of all people
4. **Importance of Human Relationships** – Social workers recognize relationships as change vehicles and engage people as partners
5. **Integrity** – Social workers behave in trustworthy manner
6. **Competence** – Social workers practice only within competence boundaries and continually enhance professional expertise

**Ethical Standards** address social workers' ethical responsibilities to clients (commitment to clients, self-determination, informed consent, competence, cultural competence, conflicts of interest, privacy and confidentiality); to colleagues (respect, confidentiality, consultation); to practice settings (supervision and consultation, education and training, performance evaluation, commitments to employers); to the profession (integrity, evaluation and research); and to society broadly (social welfare, public participation, public emergencies, social and political action).

When ethical standards conflict, the Code provides guidance: "Social workers' primary responsibility is to promote the well-being of clients. In general, clients' interests are primary. However, social workers' responsibility to the larger society or specific legal obligations may on limited occasions supersede the loyalty owed clients" (NASW, 2021, p. 7). This prioritization helps navigate tensions between individual client needs and broader social welfare but does not eliminate difficult judgment about when broader obligations override client loyalty.

# Systematic Ethical Decision-Making Frameworks

Several structured frameworks guide ethical decision-making in complex situations. While no framework eliminates difficulty, systematic approaches improve reasoning quality and consistency.

**Dolgoff, Harrington, and Loewenberg's ethical principles screen** (2012) provides hierarchical ranking when ethical principles conflict:

1. Principle of protection of life
2. Principle of equality and inequality
3. Principle of autonomy and freedom
4. Principle of least harm
5. Principle of quality of life
6. Principle of privacy and confidentiality
7. Principle of truthfulness and full disclosure

This hierarchy suggests that when principles conflict, higher-ranked principles generally take precedence. For example, protecting life (1) outweighs privacy (6), but autonomy (3) may be limited to prevent harm (4). While useful, rigid hierarchies cannot account for contextual nuances; some situations warrant flexibility.

**Congress's ETHIC model** provides mnemonic for systematic consideration:

- **E**xamine relevant values, including personal, professional, organizational, client, and societal values.
- **T**hink about what ethical standards apply, reviewing Code of Ethics and other relevant guidelines.
- **H**ypthesize different courses of action and their consequences.
- **I**dentify who will benefit and who will be harmed by each option.

- Consult with colleagues, supervisors, ethics committees, or other resources.

This framework ensures comprehensive analysis while remaining flexible about weighting different factors.

**Reamer's Guidelines for Ethical Decision-Making** (2013) emphasize:

1. Identify the ethical issues and all individuals or groups who may be affected
2. Identify all potentially relevant values, principles, and professional guidelines
3. Examine the reasons for and against each course of action, considering ethical theories, principles, and relevant codes of ethics
4. Consult with colleagues and appropriate experts
5. Make decision and document the decision-making process
6. Monitor, evaluate, and document the decision's implementation and impact

Documentation proves crucial for professional accountability and learning from experience.

# Common Ethical Dilemmas in Medical Social Work

Understanding recurring dilemma patterns enables preparation and recognition when they arise.

**End-of-life decision-making for incapacitated patients:** When patients lack capacity and advance directives, families may disagree about appropriate care. Some members may advocate for aggressive life-sustaining treatment; others prefer comfort care. Medical teams may view continued aggressive treatment as futile or harmful while families view stopping as giving up. Social workers navigate these conflicts by facilitating family communication, clarifying medical realities, exploring patient's known values, ensuring all voices are heard, involving palliative care and ethics consultation when helpful, and supporting families through difficult decisions. Ethical principles of beneficence (what helps the patient), non-maleficence (avoiding harm and suffering), autonomy (honoring patient's probable wishes), and family wellbeing all require consideration.

**Discharge to unsafe situations:** Patients sometimes face discharge to situations social workers view as unsafe: inadequate housing, absent caregiving, active substance use environments, or domestic violence. Competent patients have autonomy rights to accept risks and return to imperfect situations. However, social workers have obligations to prevent harm when possible. This dilemma involves balancing respect for autonomy with beneficence and non-maleficence. Approaches include thorough capacity assessment (ensuring patient understands risks and makes informed choice), creative problem-solving to improve safety without preventing discharge, documentation of concerns and alternatives offered, and follow-up plans to reassess after discharge.

**Resource allocation and rationing:** When social workers with limited time, attention, or resources serve multiple patients, allocation becomes necessary. Which patients receive priority? How much time should be spent on one patient when others also need service? Utilitarian frameworks suggest prioritizing patients where intervention produces most benefit. Justice frameworks emphasize equitable distribution and attention to the most vulnerable. These dilemmas lack perfect solutions but require transparent reasoning about priorities.

**Conflicts between patient needs and institutional policies:** Health care organizations establish policies for efficiency, consistency, and risk management that may conflict with individual patient needs. Examples include restrictive visitor policies that prevent important support persons, discharge protocols that prioritize bed availability over patient readiness, or insurance-driven length-of-stay pressures. Social workers must balance employment loyalty with patient advocacy. Strategies include advocating within institutional processes for policy exceptions or changes, documenting how policies harm patients, involving patient advocates or ethics committees, and in extreme cases, whistleblowing when policies create serious harm (Reamer, 2013).

**Confidentiality in family and group settings:** When providing family therapy or group interventions in medical settings, maintaining confidentiality becomes complex. What one family member shares may affect others; group members' privacy cannot be guaranteed by the social worker alone. Informed consent must address confidentiality limits in these settings, expectations must be established about what may be shared outside sessions, and social workers must navigate disclosures that create harm or risk if kept confidential versus harm if revealed.

## Moral Distress in Health Care Settings

Moral distress occurs when individuals know the ethically appropriate action but face institutional constraints, power hierarchies, or resource limitations preventing that action (Jameton, 1984). Health care providers, including social workers, frequently experience moral distress when witnessing suffering they cannot alleviate, participating in care they believe harmful, or facing institutional policies that compromise patient welfare. Unlike ethical dilemmas involving uncertainty about right action, moral distress involves certainty about what should be done but inability to act accordingly.

**Sources of moral distress for social workers:**

- inadequate resources preventing comprehensive patient support
- discharge pressure creating unsafe transitions
- witnessing aggressive end-of-life treatment causing suffering when patient's values favor comfort
- institutional policies prioritizing efficiency or profit over patient welfare
- power differentials preventing social work voices from influencing decisions
- participation in systems that perpetuate health inequities

**Consequences of moral distress:** Unaddressed moral distress contributes to burnout, compassion fatigue, job dissatisfaction, intention to leave the profession, emotional numbing, cynicism, and physical health problems (Epstein & Delgado, 2010). Organizations lose experienced practitioners; patients lose dedicated advocates; social workers lose professional fulfillment.

**Addressing moral distress:** Individual strategies include naming and acknowledging moral distress rather than dismissing it, seeking supervision and peer support to process experiences, engaging in advocacy to change distressing conditions, setting boundaries to limit exposure when possible, and utilizing employee assistance programs or therapy when distress becomes overwhelming. Organizational responses include creating ethics committees and processes for raising concerns, supporting staff through debriefing after morally distressing events, examining and addressing policies that create predictable distress, and fostering cultures where ethical concerns are welcomed rather than punished (Rushton et al., 2013).

## Utilizing Ethics Consultation and Institutional Resources

Many health care organizations provide ethics consultation services to assist with complex ethical dilemmas. Social workers should know how to access these resources and when consultation proves beneficial.

**When to seek an ethics consultation:**

- disagreement among stakeholders about goals of care or treatment decisions
- concerns about patient capacity or surrogate decision-making appropriateness
- conflicts between ethical principles without clear resolution
- questions about withdrawing or withholding life-sustaining treatment
- concerns about potential futility of interventions

- situations where legal and ethical obligations appear to conflict
- new or unusual situations without clear precedent

**Ethics consultation models:** Some institutions employ individual ethics consultants (often physicians, nurses, or social workers with ethics training). Others use ethics committees comprised of multidisciplinary professionals including physicians, nurses, social workers, chaplains, administrators, and community representatives. Consultation may involve bedside meetings with patients and families, team discussions, or formal case conferences (Fox et al., 2007).

**Social workers on ethics committees:** Social workers contribute unique perspectives to ethics committees including attention to family systems and relationships, awareness of resource and social determinants affecting decisions, cultural competence and understanding of diverse values, and commitment to social justice and equity. Social workers should pursue ethics committee involvement in their institutions when possible.

**Other institutional resources:** Patient advocates or ombudspersons address patient concerns and complaints. Risk management and legal counsel advise on legal obligations and implications. Quality improvement and patient safety committees address systemic issues. Knowing these resources and their appropriate uses strengthens ethical practice.

## Critical Thinking Questions

1. Analyze the four-principles approach (autonomy, beneficence, non-maleficence, justice) from a postcolonial or Indigenous ethics perspective. How might this framework reflect particular cultural values that are not universal? What alternative ethical frameworks might better honor diverse worldviews?
2. Evaluate the concept of moral distress in health care. How do institutional structures and power hierarchies create conditions for moral distress disproportionately affecting certain professional roles including social work, nursing, and other typically feminized professions? What organizational changes would address root causes rather than treating moral distress as individual problem?
3. Critique the social work Code of Ethics regarding its guidance when clients' interests conflict with broader social welfare. How clear is this guidance in practice? What theoretical frameworks from political philosophy or ethics might strengthen social workers' reasoning about these conflicts?
4. Examine resource allocation dilemmas through capabilities approach or other alternatives to utilitarian frameworks. How might these approaches lead to different allocation decisions? What values do different allocation frameworks privilege, and whose interests are served?

## Key Takeaways

- Ethical dilemmas involve conflicts between values, principles, or obligations without clear right answers, requiring systematic moral reasoning rather than technical problem-solving.
- Multiple ethical theories (principlism, deontology, utilitarianism, virtue ethics, care ethics, social justice) provide different lenses for analysis, each with strengths and limitations.
- The NASW Code of Ethics establishes profession-specific values and priorities, generally placing client wellbeing as primary while recognizing broader social obligations.
- Systematic decision-making frameworks improve ethical reasoning consistency and comprehensiveness through structured consideration of values, principles, stakeholders, and consequences.

- Common dilemmas include end-of-life decisions for incapacitated patients, discharges to unsafe situations, resource allocation, institutional policy conflicts, and confidentiality in family/group settings.
- Moral distress emerges when constraints prevent ethically appropriate action, contributing to burnout and requiring both individual coping and organizational response.
- Ethics consultation and institutional resources provide valuable support for complex cases, with social workers contributing unique perspectives to ethics committees.

CHAPTER 14

# Health Equity and Social Justice

## Learning Objectives

By the end of this chapter, you will be able to do the following:

- Define health equity and distinguish it from health equality
- Analyze how social determinants of health create and perpetuate health disparities
- Apply structural competency and anti-oppressive frameworks to medical social work practice
- Identify and address implicit bias and structural racism in health care systems
- Engage in individual advocacy and collective action for health equity

## Defining Health Equity and Understanding Disparities

Health equity means that everyone has a fair and just opportunity to be as healthy as possible, requiring removal of obstacles to health including poverty, discrimination, and their consequences (Braveman et al., 2011). Health equity differs fundamentally from health equality. Equality means treating everyone the same, providing identical resources and interventions regardless of need. Equity means providing resources and support matched to individual and community needs so that everyone can achieve comparable outcomes despite different starting points and barriers.

The distinction proves crucial. Providing identical diabetes education to all patients represents equality. Providing education in multiple languages, at appropriate health literacy levels, with consideration of cultural food practices, and addressing barriers like food insecurity and medication costs represents equity. Equity recognizes that different people face different barriers and require different supports to reach similar health levels.

**Health disparities** are preventable differences in disease burden, injury, violence, or opportunities to achieve optimal health experienced by socially disadvantaged populations (Braveman, 2006). These disparities manifest across multiple dimensions:

**Racial and ethnic disparities:** Compared to White Americans, Black Americans experience significantly higher rates of infant mortality (10.8 per 1,000 live births versus 4.6), maternal mortality (Black women are 3–4 times more likely to die from pregnancy-related causes), cardiovascular disease, diabetes, certain cancers, and COVID-19 mortality. Hispanic/Latino populations face higher diabetes prevalence and lower rates of cancer screening. American Indian/Alaska Native populations experience highest rates of diabetes nationally and elevated substance use disorder prevalence. Asian American and Pacific Islander populations experience disparities in liver cancer and hepatitis B (Williams & Mohammed, 2013).

These disparities persist even after controlling for socioeconomic factors, income, education, and insurance status. This persistence implicates racism and discrimination as independent causal factors beyond economic disadvantage. Weathering hypothesis research demonstrates that chronic exposure to social and economic adversity creates physiological deterioration, with stress responses including elevated blood pressure and cortisol contributing to earlier onset of chronic conditions and accelerated aging among Black Americans (Geronimus et al., 2006).

**Socioeconomic disparities:** Low-income individuals experience worse health across nearly all measures compared to higher-income individuals, with gradient effects showing that each step down the income ladder corresponds to worse health outcomes. People living in poverty face higher mortality, shorter life expectancy, greater chronic disease burden, and reduced access to preventive care and treatment. Education level similarly correlates with health; college graduates live longer and healthier lives than high school graduates, who outlive those without high school completion (Braveman et al., 2011).

**Geographic disparities:** Rural populations face higher all-cause mortality rates, limited health care access due to provider shortages, greater distances to specialized care, and reduced availability of mental health and substance use treatment services. Urban-rural disparities affect preventive care utilization, cancer mortality, maternal health outcomes, and chronic disease management. Within urban areas, neighborhood-level disparities create dramatic health outcome differences across zip codes in the same city, with some neighborhoods experiencing life expectancies 20+ years shorter than affluent neighborhoods just miles away (Singh & Siahpush, 2014).

**Gender and sexual orientation disparities:** Women face unique health challenges including maternal mortality disparities (Black women are 3–4 times more likely to die from pregnancy-related causes than White women) and higher rates of certain chronic conditions. Sexual and gender minority populations experience elevated rates of mental health conditions, substance use, violence victimization, and suicide attempts, partly attributable to minority stress from discrimination and stigma. Transgender individuals face profound health care access barriers including insurance denials, provider discrimination, lack of provider knowledge, and violence (Stanton, 2020).

**Disability-related disparities:** People with disabilities experience higher rates of obesity, smoking, physical inactivity, and inadequate preventive care. They encounter communication barriers, physical accessibility barriers in health care facilities, provider attitudinal barriers, and discrimination in treatment decisions. Health care systems often fail to provide reasonable accommodations required by law, creating access barriers for populations already experiencing health vulnerabilities (Krahn et al., 2015).

These disparities are not random, natural, or inevitable. They result from social determinants of health shaped by unjust social structures, discriminatory policies, and ongoing oppression.

## Social Determinants of Health Framework

Social determinants of health (SDOH) are conditions in environments where people are born, live, learn, work, play, worship, and age that affect health, functioning, and quality of life outcomes and risks (Healthy People 2030). The SDOH framework fundamentally shifts focus from individual behavior change and personal responsibility narratives to structural factors shaping health opportunities and outcomes.

**Healthy People 2030 identifies five key SDOH domains:**

1. **Economic stability** encompasses employment status, income level, expenses and debt, medical bills, and financial support systems. Poverty creates chronic stress, limits access to healthy food and safe housing, prevents health care utilization due to cost, and correlates with virtually all negative health outcomes. Economic instability affects not only material resources but also psychological wellbeing through chronic uncertainty and worry. Research demonstrates dose-response relationships; each incremental increase in income corresponds to improved health outcomes across the income distribution, not merely comparing poverty to affluence (Braveman et al., 2011).
2. **Education access and quality** includes early childhood education and development, enrollment in higher education, high school graduation rates, language and literacy, and educational support.

Education strongly predicts health through multiple pathways including better employment opportunities and income, health literacy enabling informed health decisions, social networks and support, sense of control and self-efficacy, and cognitive functioning. Educational experiences in childhood and adolescence shape health trajectories across the lifespan. Educational inequity perpetuates health inequity generationally (Zajacova & Lawrence, 2018).

3. **Health care access and quality** addresses health insurance coverage, provider availability and accessibility, provider cultural and linguistic competency, quality of care received, and health literacy. While health care represents just one social determinant among many (non-medical factors prove more influential for population health than medical care), access affects screening and early detection, chronic disease management, acute care during illness, and preventive services. Uninsured and underinsured individuals delay care, experience worse health outcomes, and face medical debt creating financial instability that compounds health problems.
4. **Neighborhood and built environment** encompasses housing quality, access to transportation, availability of healthy foods, walkability and opportunities for physical activity, air and water quality, neighborhood crime and violence, and environmental exposures. Living in disadvantaged neighborhoods independently predicts poor health outcomes through multiple mechanisms including exposure to violence and chronic stress, environmental toxins and pollutants, limited access to healthy food (food deserts), unsafe conditions preventing physical activity, and inadequate housing quality (Diez Roux & Mair, 2010). Residential segregation, a product of discriminatory policies, concentrates these neighborhood disadvantages in communities of color.
5. **Social and community context** includes social cohesion, civic participation, perceptions of discrimination and equity, incarceration rates, and social support networks. Strong social connections and community cohesion protect health through instrumental support, emotional support, sense of belonging, and collective efficacy. Conversely, discrimination creates chronic stress with documented physiological impacts, social isolation increases mortality risk, and mass incarceration disrupts families and communities while creating lasting health harms (Williams & Mohammed, 2013).

**Upstream factors:** Beyond individual-level SDOH, structural factors shape SDOH distribution including systemic racism, economic policies creating inequality, residential segregation, educational funding mechanisms perpetuating inequality, political structures affecting representation and power, and climate change disproportionately affecting marginalized communities. Addressing health equity requires attention to these root causes, not merely addressing proximal determinants (Williams et al., 2019).

## Structural Racism as Fundamental Cause of Health Inequities

While multiple factors contribute to health disparities, structural racism represents a fundamental cause producing racial health inequities through multiple mechanisms (Bailey et al., 2017). Structural racism refers to macro-level systems, social forces, institutions, ideologies, and processes that generate and reinforce inequities among racial and ethnic groups. Unlike individual prejudice or interpersonal discrimination, structural racism operates through policies, practices, and norms embedded in institutions.

### Historical Context

Current racial health disparities connect directly to historical injustices including slavery's brutal health impacts, genocide and forced removal of Indigenous peoples, exclusion from property ownership and wealth accumulation, segregation legally mandating unequal treatment, discriminatory New Deal and GI Bill policies creating wealth disparities, medical experimentation without consent (Tuskegee Syphilis Study, forced sterilization), and redlining concentrating poverty and limiting investment in communities of color. These historical harms created wealth gaps, educational disparities, and residential segregation that persist and compound across generations (Bailey et al., 2017).

The United States has never addressed these historical harms through reparations, truth and reconciliation, or comprehensive policy remediation. Instead, contemporary policies and practices continue producing racial inequities while maintaining plausible deniability through facially race-neutral language that produces racially disparate impacts.

## Mechanisms of Structural Racism in Health Care

1. **Residential segregation:** Policies including redlining (Federal Housing Administration refusing to insure mortgages in Black neighborhoods), discriminatory lending practices, restrictive covenants, exclusionary zoning, and highway construction through communities of color created profound residential segregation. This segregation concentrates poverty, limits wealth accumulation through home ownership, creates environmental health hazards, reduces tax base affecting school quality, limits access to healthy food and quality health care, and exposes residents to violence and chronic stress. Residential segregation represents perhaps the most powerful mechanism through which structural racism produces health inequities (Williams & Collins, 2001).
2. **Educational inequity:** School funding based on property taxes perpetuates inequality, with segregated schools in low-wealth communities receiving inadequate resources. Differential educational quality limits health literacy, future employment and income, and opportunities throughout life. Discriminatory discipline practices and low expectations for students of color create additional barriers.
3. **Employment discrimination and occupational segregation:** Discrimination in hiring, promotion, and pay concentrate people of color in jobs with greater physical hazards, lower pay, limited benefits including health insurance, less job security, and fewer opportunities for advancement. Occupational segregation affects income, exposure to occupational hazards, access to employer-sponsored insurance, and economic stability.
4. **Criminal justice system:** Mass incarceration disproportionately affecting Black and Latino communities creates profound health impacts. Incarceration disrupts families, creates trauma, limits future employment through criminal records, disenfranchises individuals affecting political power, and directly harms health through inadequate health care in prisons and jails and exposure to violence. The War on Drugs created racially disparate incarceration despite similar drug use rates across racial groups (Wildeman & Wang, 2017).
5. **Health care system discrimination:** Evidence documents differential treatment quality within health care, with patients of color receiving less adequate pain management, fewer referrals to specialists, lower quality cardiac care, less aggressive cancer treatment, and systematically different care even when insurance status, income, and other factors are controlled. This differential treatment reflects provider implicit bias, structural barriers within health care organizations, and medical mistrust developed through historical and ongoing mistreatment (Institute of Medicine, 2003).
6. **Weathering:** Chronic exposure to social and economic adversity and political marginalization creates physiological deterioration through stress pathways. Research demonstrates that Black Americans experience higher allostatic load (cumulative physiological wear and tear from chronic stress) at younger ages compared to White Americans, contributing to earlier onset of chronic conditions, premature aging, and shorter life expectancy. This weathering effect represents biological embedding of social inequality (Geronimus et al., 2006).
7. **Social work response to structural racism:** Addressing structural racism requires moving beyond individual cultural competence training to structural competency, anti-racist practice, and collective action for systemic change. These include the following:

- explicitly acknowledging racism's role in creating and maintaining health disparities rather than attributing disparities to genetics, culture, or individual behavior
- examining how one's own professional practice may inadvertently perpetuate racist structures even with good intentions
- centering voices and leadership of communities of color in research, practice, and policy development
- advocating for policies addressing root causes including residential segregation, educational inequity, and criminal justice reform
- building coalitions across disciplines and with community organizations for systemic change
- committing to ongoing learning, critical self-reflection, and action rather than treating anti-racism as completed training

# Structural Competency and Anti-Oppressive Practice

**Structural competency** extends cultural competence frameworks by training practitioners to recognize and address structural factors including racism, poverty, immigration policies, and systemic barriers that produce health inequities (Metzl & Hansen, 2014). Rather than attributing health disparities primarily to individual behaviors or cultural differences, structural competency emphasizes how institutions, policies, and social structures shape health outcomes.

**Five core competencies include the following:**

1. **Recognizing structures shaping clinical interactions:** Understanding how housing policies, neighborhood disinvestment, employment discrimination, and institutional practices influence health problems rather than attributing everything to individual choices or cultural factors. For example, recognizing that a patient's difficulty managing diabetes reflects food insecurity created by poverty wages and food deserts rather than cultural food preferences or noncompliance.
2. **Developing structural humility:** Acknowledging limits of individual clinical interventions when structural barriers exist and recognizing need for systemic change alongside individual support. Clinical excellence cannot overcome unjust structures; health equity requires structural transformation.
3. **Rearticulating cultural formulations in structural terms:** Moving beyond cultural explanations to examine how structural racism, economic oppression, and immigration policy create patterns that might be attributed to culture. For instance, recognizing that mistrust of health care institutions among Black patients reflects rational responses to historical and ongoing discrimination rather than cultural paranoia.
4. **Observing and imagining structural interventions:** Identifying opportunities for advocacy, policy change, and collective action to address root causes. This includes recognizing when problems presented as individual clinical issues require structural responses.
5. **Developing structural reflexivity:** Examining how one's own position within health care systems and broader society shapes perspectives, creates blind spots regarding structural factors, and may contribute to perpetuating inequities despite good intentions.

**Anti-oppressive practice** represents a social work framework explicitly addressing power, privilege, and oppression in all practice dimensions (Baines, 2017). Core principles include the following:

1. **Centering marginalized voices:** Ensuring that research, practice, and policy development center leadership and expertise of communities most affected by inequities rather than professionals speaking for communities. This includes participatory approaches, community-based participatory research, and deferring to community priorities.
2. **Examining power dynamics:** Analyzing power relations in professional-client relationships, orga-

nizational hierarchies, and broader social structures. Anti-oppressive practice acknowledges that social workers hold professional power and institutional authority that may be experienced as oppressive regardless of good intentions.

3. **Challenging dominant narratives:** Questioning mainstream explanations that blame individuals or cultures for problems created by structural oppression. This includes challenging deficit-based language, pathologizing narratives, and cultural explanations that obscure structural causes.
4. **Reflexivity about practitioner position:** Continuous examination of how one's own race, class, gender, ability, and other social locations shape perspectives, interactions, and blind spots. This involves discomfort, ongoing learning, and willingness to be challenged.
5. **Advocacy for systemic change:** Recognizing that individual interventions prove insufficient without structural transformation. Anti-oppressive practice includes advocacy, policy work, and collective action alongside clinical services.
6. **Solidarity and allyship:** Developing authentic relationships and partnerships with communities and movements for social justice, using professional privilege and resources in service of community-led change efforts.

Anti-oppressive practice requires ongoing discomfort, learning, and growth as practitioners confront complicity in oppressive systems while working toward transformation. It represents lifelong commitment rather than achieved competency.

# Individual and Collective Advocacy for Health Equity

Social workers engage in health equity advocacy at multiple levels from individual case advocacy to policy change and community organizing.

**Case advocacy** addresses barriers facing individual patients:

- appealing insurance denials for medically necessary services
- connecting patients to financial assistance, food programs, housing resources, and transportation
- advocating with health care teams for appropriate, non-discriminatory care
- challenging stigmatizing language or assumptions about patients
- ensuring language access through professional interpretation
- requesting reasonable accommodations for patients with disabilities
- documenting social determinants and their health impacts

While essential, case advocacy alone cannot eliminate structural barriers affecting multiple patients. Individual solutions to systemic problems prove inadequate for achieving health equity.

**Organizational Advocacy** works within institutions to change policies, practices, and cultures perpetuating inequity:

- participating in committees addressing health equity, quality improvement, or patient experience
- proposing policy changes reducing barriers (visitor policies, financial assistance criteria, discharge protocols)
- providing staff training on structural competency, trauma-informed care, and anti-bias
- supporting diverse workforce recruitment and retention
- advocating for language access services and culturally appropriate materials
- collecting and analyzing data revealing disparities to drive improvement
- challenging institutional practices that discriminate or disadvantage vulnerable populations

Social workers' positions within organizations enable insider advocacy, though this may create tensions with employment loyalty and power dynamics.

**Legislative and policy advocacy** influences laws and policies shaping health and health care:

- Medicaid expansion ensuring coverage for low-income individuals
- insurance coverage requirements preventing discrimination
- housing policy including affordable housing development and tenant protections
- living wage laws and worker protections
- environmental regulations addressing pollution in marginalized communities
- criminal justice reform reducing mass incarceration's health impacts
- immigration policy affecting health care access

Strategies include educating legislators through meetings and written materials, testifying at hearings, mobilizing constituents to contact representatives, joining advocacy coalitions, using media to raise awareness, and participating in electoral politics. NASW maintains active policy advocacy infrastructure that members can amplify.

**Community organizing and coalition building** partners with affected communities leading change efforts:

- following community leadership and priorities rather than imposing professional agendas
- building long-term authentic relationships beyond project timelines
- sharing resources, information, and professional privilege
- supporting community-defined strategies and goals
- participating in coalitions addressing health equity, housing justice, economic justice, and racial justice
- contributing professional expertise while learning from community wisdom

Authentic partnership requires humility, power-sharing, and sustained commitment.

**Research and knowledge production** documents disparities, evaluates interventions, and amplifies community narratives:

- conducting research on health inequities and their causes
- evaluating interventions and policies for equity impacts
- partnering with communities in participatory action research
- translating research findings for public audiences
- challenging research that pathologizes communities or ignores structural factors
- supporting community-led research and evaluation

Social workers can conduct research, support community research, and ensure that knowledge production serves justice rather than perpetuating oppression.

## Health Equity in Daily Practice

Beyond formal advocacy, medical social workers promote health equity through daily practice decisions:

1. **Universal SDOH Screening:** Systematically assessing food security, housing stability, transportation access, utility needs, legal concerns, intimate partner violence, and other social needs for all patients rather than making assumptions based on demographics. Validated screening tools include Protocol for Responding to and Assessing Patients' Assets, Risks, and Experiences (PRAPARE) and the Accountable Health Communities screening tool. Screening identifies needs enabling intervention.

2. **Resource navigation and connection:** Maintaining comprehensive updated knowledge of community resources, establishing relationships facilitating referrals, making warm handoffs rather than simply providing lists, addressing barriers to resource access, and following up ensuring connections occurred. Resources addressing food insecurity, housing instability, utility assistance, transportation, legal aid, and other social determinants directly improve health.
3. **Equity-focused documentation:** Recording social determinants, structural barriers, discrimination observed, and advocacy undertaken creates data supporting resource allocation and systemic change. Documentation should avoid deficit language blaming patients while clearly articulating how structural factors affect health. For example, documenting housing instability and food insecurity rather than noncompliance, or noting that a patient experiences discrimination rather than labeling the patient as difficult.
4. **Culturally and linguistically appropriate services:** Implementing National CLAS Standards including providing language assistance at no cost, recruiting diverse workforce, engaging community in service design, conducting organizational self-assessment, and maintaining culturally appropriate health education materials (Office of Minority Health, 2013). Social workers should champion CLAS implementation within organizations.
5. **Addressing implicit bias:** Remaining vigilant about bias affecting clinical judgments, using structured decision-making tools reducing bias influence, seeking peer consultation when uncomfortable reactions arise, examining differential service provision across patient populations, and building authentic relationships with diverse communities reducing stereotyping through meaningful contact.
6. **Speaking up about inequities:** Naming when systems, policies, or team dynamics perpetuate inequity even when uncomfortable. This includes challenging dismissive comments about patients, questioning policies disproportionately affecting vulnerable populations, advocating for resources benefiting marginalized patients, and raising concerns about discriminatory practices. Speaking up represents ethical obligation despite potential professional costs.

## Critical Thinking Questions

1. Analyze the social determinants of health framework through a critical political economy lens. While SDOH frameworks expand focus beyond individual behavior, how might they still inadequately address power relations, capitalism, and structural violence? What theoretical frameworks from critical race theory, Indigenous scholarship, or Marxist analysis might strengthen understanding of health inequity's root causes?
2. Evaluate the concept of "health equity" versus more radical formulations like "health justice" or "health liberation." How do these different framings shape what interventions are imagined, what transformations are deemed necessary, and who holds power in defining problems and solutions? What are the political implications of choosing particular terminology?

## Key Takeaways

- Health equity means everyone has fair opportunity to be healthy, requiring removal of obstacles including poverty and discrimination; equity differs from equality by providing differential support matched to need.
- Health disparities across race, ethnicity, SES, geography, gender, sexual orientation, and disability result from social determinants shaped by unjust structures, not individual failings.
- Social determinants include economic stability, education, health care access, neighborhood environment, and social context, with upstream factors including structural racism and economic policy.

- Structural racism operates through residential segregation, educational inequity, employment discrimination, criminal justice, health care discrimination, and weathering, creating fundamental cause of racial health inequities.

CHAPTER 15

# Understanding Healthcare Laws and Policies

## Learning Objectives

By the end of this chapter, you will be able to do the following:

- Explain key federal health care laws affecting social work practice and patient rights
- Apply legal knowledge to protect patient rights and navigate system barriers
- Distinguish between legal requirements and ethical obligations when they conflict
- Utilize legal frameworks for advocacy and systems change
- Maintain current awareness of evolving health care law and policy

## Health Care Law as Social Work Competency

Legal knowledge represents essential social work competency, not because social workers serve as lawyers but because understanding legal frameworks enables effective advocacy, protects patient rights, prevents liability, and identifies where laws themselves create or perpetuate injustice (Reamer, 2013). Medical social workers regularly encounter situations where legal knowledge proves crucial: determining whether patients can refuse treatment, understanding privacy obligations, knowing when involuntary psychiatric holds are legally appropriate, accessing legal protections for patients with disabilities, and navigating complex insurance regulations.

Legal literacy strengthens practice through multiple mechanisms. First, it enables social workers to inform patients and families about legal rights, supporting informed decision-making and self-advocacy. Second, it provides frameworks for challenging institutional practices violating legal protections. Third, it clarifies professional obligations including mandated reporting and confidentiality boundaries. Fourth, it reduces liability risk by ensuring practice aligns with legal requirements. Fifth, it reveals how laws create structural barriers and inequities, informing advocacy for legal reform.

However, legal compliance alone proves insufficient for ethical practice. Laws establish minimum acceptable conduct, not aspirational standards. Ethical obligations may exceed legal requirements. Sometimes actions that are legal prove unethical, and vice versa. Social workers must navigate tensions between legal obligations and ethical commitments, using professional judgment and supervision to chart appropriate courses when law and ethics conflict (Reamer, 2013).

# HIPAA: Privacy and Confidentiality in Health Care

The Health Insurance Portability and Accountability Act of 1996 (HIPAA) establishes national standards protecting privacy and security of health information. While HIPAA is frequently invoked and commonly misunderstood, clear understanding enables appropriate information sharing while protecting patient privacy (U.S. Department of Health and Human Services, 2003).

## Protected Health Information (PHI)

HIPAA protects "individually identifiable health information" including demographic data (name, address, birth date, Social Security number, medical record number, photographs), medical information (diagnosis, treatment records, test results, clinical notes), and payment information (billing records, insurance information). Protection applies regardless of format: written, electronic, or oral communication.

## Permitted Uses and Disclosures

HIPAA permits health care providers to use and disclose PHI without patient authorization for treatment, payment, and health care operations (TPO). **Treatment** includes coordination among providers, referrals, and consultations. **Payment** encompasses billing, insurance claims, and collection activities. **Health care operations** include quality improvement, training, accreditation, business planning, and customer service.

This means social workers may share patient information with physicians involved in care, hospital billing departments, quality improvement committees, and case managers coordinating discharge without obtaining specific patient consent. However, professional ethics may require more restrictive information sharing even when HIPAA permits disclosure. The minimum necessary standard requires using or disclosing only the minimum PHI necessary to accomplish the intended purpose.

## Required Patient Rights

HIPAA grants patients specific rights:

- **Right to access:** Inspect and obtain copies of health records with limited exceptions
- **Right to amend:** Request corrections to records, though providers may deny if they believe records are accurate
- **Right to accounting:** Receive list of certain disclosures made (excluding TPO disclosures)
- **Right to restrict:** Request limitations on uses and disclosures, though providers may decline
- **Right to confidential communications:** Request communications through alternative means (different phone number, address)
- **Right to notice:** Receive Notice of Privacy Practices explaining information use and patient rights

## Permitted Disclosures Without Authorization

Beyond TPO, HIPAA permits disclosure without patient authorization in specific circumstances:

- required by law (mandated abuse reporting, court orders, public health reporting)
- public health activities (disease reporting, vaccine monitoring, FDA oversight)
- abuse, neglect, or domestic violence reporting when mandated by law
- health oversight activities (audits, investigations by health agencies)
- judicial and administrative proceedings (court orders meeting specific criteria, subpoenas with patient authorization or qualifying statements)

- law enforcement purposes (identifying suspects under limited circumstances, reporting gunshot wounds where required)
- coroners, medical examiners, funeral directors for death investigation and funeral arrangements
- organ donation purposes
- research (with specific protections and approvals)
- serious threat to health or safety when disclosure is necessary to prevent or lessen imminent threat

### Common HIPAA Misunderstandings

HIPAA does not prohibit all family communication. Providers may share information with family members, friends, or others involved in care when the patient agrees, has opportunity to object and doesn't, or when professional judgment indicates disclosure is in patient's best interest and patient is incapacitated.

HIPAA does not prevent leaving voicemail messages. Providers may leave messages but should limit information and be discreet.

HIPAA does not override stronger state privacy laws. When state laws provide greater protection, state law prevails.

HIPAA does not apply to all entities. Only covered entities (health plans, health care clearinghouses, health care providers who transmit health information electronically) and their business associates must comply. Many community organizations, employers, and schools are not HIPAA-covered.

### Intersection With Social Work Ethics

NASW Code of Ethics establishes confidentiality standards potentially exceeding HIPAA. Ethical standards require protecting client privacy beyond legal minimums. When HIPAA permits disclosure but ethics suggest withholding information, social workers should follow the more restrictive standard. Consultation with supervisors, privacy officers, or legal counsel assists navigation when uncertainty exists about appropriate disclosure.

## EMTALA: Emergency Treatment and Patient Dumping

The Emergency Medical Treatment and Active Labor Act (EMTALA; 1986) requires Medicare-participating hospitals with emergency departments to provide medical screening examination and stabilization to anyone presenting, regardless of ability to pay. EMTALA emerged in response to "patient dumping," where hospitals transferred uninsured patients to public hospitals without stabilizing conditions (Zibulewsky, 2001).

### EMTALA Key Provisions

**Medical screening examination (MSE):** Hospitals must provide an MSE to determine whether emergency medical condition exists for anyone requesting examination or treatment in the emergency department. The MSE must be provided by qualified personnel (typically physicians or mid-level providers) within the capability of the facility's emergency department and cannot be delayed to inquire about insurance or payment ability. Refusing to screen, providing cursory examinations to avoid obligations, or requiring payment before screening violates EMTALA.

**Emergency medical condition:** EMTALA defines this broadly as conditions manifesting acute symptoms of sufficient severity that absence of immediate medical attention could reasonably be expected to result in serious jeopardy to health, serious impairment to bodily functions, or serious dysfunction of bodily organs. This includes active labor in pregnant women.

**Stabilization requirement:** If an emergency medical condition exists, hospitals must provide treatment stabilizing the condition before discharge or transfer, unless the patient requests a transfer in writing after being informed of risks and benefits or a physician certifies that the medical benefits of a transfer to another facility outweigh the risks. Stabilization means providing treatment such that no material deterioration of condition is likely during or as a result of a transfer.

**Appropriate transfer:** When hospitals lack the capability to treat conditions, transfers to facilities with appropriate capability are required. However, transfers must meet specific conditions:

- receiving facility has available space and qualified personnel and agrees to accept transfer
- transferring hospital provides medical treatment within capacity minimizing transfer risks
- transfer occurs with qualified personnel and appropriate medical equipment
- copies of medical records accompany the patient
- physician certifies that benefits outweigh risks, or patient requests transfer

### Social Work Implications

Social workers should understand EMTALA protections to inform patients who fear denial of emergency care due to lack of insurance or immigration status. EMTALA ensures emergency treatment regardless of payment ability. However, EMTALA does not require ongoing treatment after stabilization. Hospitals may discharge uninsured patients once the patient is medically stable, even when continued care remains necessary.

Social workers assist with post-stabilization planning to ensure access to follow-up care, connecting patients to federally qualified health centers, charity care programs, Medicaid enrollment, and community resources. EMTALA violations should be reported to Centers for Medicare & Medicaid Services, state health departments, or hospital compliance officers.

Advocacy may be necessary when hospitals pressure premature discharge of stabilized patients based on insurance status, particularly affecting uninsured, underinsured, or undocumented individuals. Documentation of medical instability and social worker concerns protects patients and creates records supporting advocacy.

## Americans with Disabilities Act: Equal Access and Accommodation

The Americans with Disabilities Act (ADA; 1990) prohibits discrimination based on disability in employment, public services, public accommodations, and telecommunications. Health care applications prove particularly relevant for medical social workers (U.S. Department of Justice, 2010).

### Definition of Disability

The ADA defines disability broadly as physical or mental impairment substantially limiting one or more major life activities, record of such impairment, or being regarded as having impairment. Major life activities include caring for oneself, performing manual tasks, seeing, hearing, eating, sleeping, walking, standing, sitting, reaching, lifting, bending, speaking, breathing, learning, reading, concentrating, thinking, communicating, interacting with others, and working. Major bodily functions including immune system, cardiovascular, neurological, respiratory, and reproductive functions also constitute major life activities.

Conditions covered include but are not limited to mobility impairments, blindness and visual impairments, deafness and hearing impairments, speech impairments, intellectual disabilities, autism spectrum disorders, psychiatric disabilities (depression, PTSD, schizophrenia, bipolar disorder), chronic illnesses (diabetes, cancer, multiple sclerosis, HIV/AIDS), and temporary substantial impairments.

## Title II: Public Services

Government-operated health care facilities including public hospitals, health departments, and state psychiatric hospitals must ensure services, programs, and activities are accessible to people with disabilities. Requirements include

- physical accessibility of buildings and facilities
- effective communication through auxiliary aids and services
- program modifications unless fundamental alteration or undue burden
- prohibition of disability-based discrimination in service provision

## Title III: Public Accommodations

Private health care providers including hospitals, clinics, doctor's offices, pharmacies, and medical offices constitute public accommodations and must remove barriers to access. Requirements include

- accessible physical spaces (ramps, automatic doors, accessible exam tables and equipment, accessible restrooms)
- effective communication (qualified interpreters, assistive listening devices, accessible formats for medical information)
- service animal accommodation in all areas patients are allowed
- prohibition of disability-based discrimination including in service provision, treatment allocation, and insurance

**Effective communication:** Health care providers must ensure effective communication with patients and companions with disabilities affecting hearing, vision, or speech. For deaf or hard of hearing individuals, this typically requires qualified sign language interpreters for substantive medical discussions including diagnosis, prognosis, treatment options, consent, and discharge instructions. "Qualified" means interpreters possess specialized medical vocabulary, training, and certification. Family members, particularly children, are inadequate and inappropriate substitutes except in true emergencies.

For blind or low vision individuals, providers must offer materials in Braille, large print, audio formats, or electronic formats compatible with screen readers. For individuals with speech disabilities, providers must exercise patience, allow extra time, use appropriate communication methods, and avoid making assumptions about cognitive capacity based on speech differences.

**Reasonable modifications:** Providers must modify policies, practices, and procedures when necessary unless modifications would fundamentally alter services or create undue burden. Examples include

- allowing service animals in all patient areas including operating rooms when feasible
- providing extra appointment time for patients requiring additional communication or mobility assistance
- permitting companions to remain with patients who need assistance
- modifying usual procedures to accommodate cognitive or psychiatric disabilities
- allowing patients to bring necessary disability-related equipment

## Social Work Advocacy

Medical social workers ensure disability rights are respected by

- requesting professional interpreters and accessibility accommodations proactively
- educating patients about ADA rights and how to request accommodations

- challenging discriminatory practices, assumptions about quality of life with disabilities, or communication with caregivers rather than patients
- ensuring discharge planning considers disability-related needs and home modifications
- advocating for organizational ADA compliance including staff training
- addressing common violations: failing to provide interpreters, assuming patients with intellectual disabilities cannot participate in decisions, making decisions with family rather than the patient who has disability, physical inaccessibility, and discrimination in treatment decisions

## Mental Health Laws: Involuntary Commitment and Patient Rights

State mental health laws govern involuntary psychiatric holds, commitment procedures, and rights of individuals receiving mental health treatment. While laws vary by state, common elements exist across jurisdictions. Medical social workers regularly encounter situations requiring mental health law knowledge including suicidal or homicidal patients, severe psychiatric symptoms impairing function or safety, and patients refusing voluntary psychiatric care (Anfang & Appelbaum, 2006).

### Emergency Psychiatric Holds

All states provide mechanisms for short-term involuntary psychiatric evaluation when individuals meet specific criteria. Common criteria include the following.

- **Danger to self:** Suicidal ideation with intent and plan, self-harm behaviors, severe neglect of basic needs creating imminent health risk
- **Danger to others:** Homicidal or violent ideation with identifiable victims, recent violent behavior, threats creating reasonable fear
- **Gravely disabled:** Unable to provide for basic needs (food, clothing, shelter) due to mental illness, creating imminent danger

Hold durations vary by state (typically 72 hours to 14 days) and require physician or designated mental health professional certification. Patients retain rights during holds including humane treatment, freedom from unnecessary restraint, communication with attorneys and designated contacts, and judicial review. Some states permit law enforcement to initiate holds; others require medical professional determination.

### Civil Commitment

Extended involuntary treatment beyond emergency holds requires judicial proceedings with higher evidentiary standards. Typical requirements include

- clear and convincing evidence (higher than preponderance but lower than beyond reasonable doubt) that patient meets commitment criteria
- demonstration that patient has serious mental illness
- proof that less restrictive alternatives are inappropriate or inadequate
- evidence that voluntary treatment has been offered and refused or tried and failed

Patients have due process rights including written notice of proceedings, judicial hearing within specified timeframes, legal representation (often court-appointed if patient cannot afford attorney), ability to present evidence and call witnesses, right to cross-examine witnesses, and right to appeal. Commitment orders specify maximum treatment duration and conditions, with periodic review required.

## Outpatient Commitment

Approximately 47 states allow court-ordered outpatient treatment (assisted outpatient treatment or AOT) for individuals with serious mental illness meeting specific criteria beyond dangerousness, typically including treatment non-adherence history, deterioration pattern, and likelihood of benefiting from outpatient treatment. Outpatient commitment aims to prevent hospitalization through mandated medication and treatment adherence.

Controversy exists regarding outpatient commitment effectiveness and ethics. Proponents cite reduced hospitalization and homelessness in some studies. Critics raise concerns about coercion, civil liberties, discrimination, and whether coerced treatment produces genuine therapeutic benefits. Social workers should understand their state's outpatient commitment laws and critically examine both potential benefits and risks.

## Patient Rights in Psychiatric Settings

Even when involuntarily hospitalized, patients retain fundamental rights:

- treatment in least restrictive setting appropriate to clinical needs
- individualized treatment plan with patient participation when possible
- periodic review of continued hospitalization necessity
- freedom from restraint and seclusion except when clinically necessary to prevent imminent harm
- right to refuse treatment (with judicial override possible in some circumstances after hearings)
- privacy and confidentiality protections
- communication access including phone calls and visitors (with reasonable restrictions)
- grievance procedures for addressing concerns
- humane treatment conditions and protection from abuse

Social workers advocate for these rights, help patients understand and exercise them, investigate rights violations, and support patients through complaint processes.

## Capacity and Competency

Mental illness does not automatically render individuals incompetent or lacking in a decision-making capacity. Psychiatric patients retain autonomy and decision-making rights unless specifically found to lack capacity for particular decisions through appropriate assessment. Social workers ensure that capacity is assessed appropriately rather than assumed based on diagnosis, psychiatric hospitalization status, or unconventional beliefs.

## Tarasoff Duty

Following *Tarasoff v. Regents of the University of California* (1976), most states have imposed a duty to protect third parties when mental health professionals determine that patients pose serious danger to identifiable individuals. This duty may require warning the threatened individual, notifying law enforcement, or involuntarily hospitalizing the patient. Specific requirements vary by state, with some states requiring warning (duty to warn) and others permitting various protective actions (duty to protect).

Social workers must understand their state's specific Tarasoff provisions including who is covered (all mental health professionals vs. specific licenses), what triggers the duty (serious threat vs. any threat, identifiable vs. general threats), and what actions satisfy the duty (warning victim, notifying police, hospitalization). Consultation with supervisors and legal counsel assists navigation when situations potentially triggering duty arise.

### Social Work Considerations

Involuntary psychiatric treatment creates profound ethical tensions between beneficence (helping individuals who may not recognize need for treatment), protection (preventing harm to self or others), and autonomy (respecting self-determination even when choices appear unwise). Social workers should

- exhaust voluntary treatment options before pursuing involuntary interventions
- minimize coercion and maximize choice within legal constraints
- ensure holds meet legal criteria and are not inappropriately used for social problems, homelessness, or substance use without mental illness
- advocate for least restrictive alternatives to hospitalization when clinically appropriate
- attend to racial and other disparities in involuntary treatment reflecting systemic biases
- support patients' rights during and after involuntary treatment
- document thoroughly the basis for believing legal criteria are met

Research documents racial disparities with Black individuals experiencing higher rates of involuntary hospitalization, seclusion, and restraint compared to White individuals with similar clinical presentations. These disparities reflect implicit bias, structural racism in mental health systems, and broader social factors creating disproportionate police involvement with Black individuals experiencing mental health crises. Social workers must acknowledge and work to address these inequities (Lindsey et al., 2010).

## Health Care Policy and Advocacy

Beyond understanding specific laws, social workers engage with health care policy shaping system structure, coverage, access, and equity. Major policy areas include:

### Insurance Coverage Policy

Medicaid expansion under the Affordable Care Act (ACA) extended coverage to millions, reducing uninsurance rates and improving access. However, 10 states have not expanded Medicaid, creating coverage gaps. Medicare coverage policies determine what services are reimbursed and under what conditions. Private insurance regulation addresses essential health benefits, pre-existing condition protections, and lifetime/annual coverage limits. The Children's Health Insurance Program (CHIP) covers children in families with incomes too high for Medicaid but too low for affordable private insurance.

Social work advocacy involves supporting Medicaid expansion in non-expansion states, protecting ACA provisions from repeal efforts, advocating for public option or single-payer systems, addressing coverage gaps in current systems, and supporting safety net programs serving uninsured and underinsured populations.

### Reimbursement Policy

Medicare and Medicaid reimbursement rates affect provider availability, service delivery models, and access to care. Low reimbursement rates create provider shortages in some specialties and geographic areas. Payment models including fee-for-service, capitation, bundled payments, and value-based purchasing shape care delivery. Social work advocacy addresses

- recognition and reimbursement for social work services across settings
- payment models supporting integrated behavioral health and medical care
- adequate rates ensuring access for Medicaid beneficiaries
- alternative payment models rewarding quality and outcomes rather than volume

## Mental Health and Addiction Parity

The Mental Health Parity and Addiction Equity Act (MHPAEA, 2008) requires insurance plans to cover mental health and substance use disorder (MH/SUD) treatment at parity with medical/surgical coverage. Plans cannot impose more restrictive limitations on MH/SUD benefits including higher co-pays, stricter visit limits, or more stringent authorization requirements.

However, parity implementation and enforcement remain incomplete. Plans use narrow networks, aggressive utilization review, and medical necessity denials creating de facto limitations despite parity requirements. Social workers advocate for meaningful parity enforcement, help patients file complaints when parity is violated, and support legislative strengthening of parity requirements.

## Health Care Civil Rights

Title VI of the Civil Rights Act prohibits discrimination based on race, color, or national origin in federally funded programs, requiring language access and culturally appropriate services. Section 1557 of the ACA extends protections based on sex, including protections for LGBTQ+ individuals and the prohibition of denial of gender-affirming care coverage and services for transgender individuals. Social workers monitor implementation, advocate when violations occur, and educate patients about civil rights protections.

## Public Health and Social Determinants Policy

While typically not considered "health care policy," policies addressing social determinants profoundly affect health and health equity:

- housing policy (affordable housing development, eviction protections, lead abatement, housing quality standards)
- nutrition policy (SNAP, WIC, school meals, food security programs)
- environmental policy (air and water quality, toxic exposure prevention, climate change mitigation)
- education policy (school funding, early childhood programs, higher education access)
- economic policy (minimum wage, paid sick leave, unemployment insurance, tax policy)

Social workers bring health perspective to these broader policy areas, documenting health impacts of policies, advocating for health-promoting policies, and building coalitions across sectors.

## Policy Advocacy Strategies

Social workers engage in policy advocacy through multiple avenues:

- educating legislators through meetings, letters, emails, and phone calls
- providing testimony at legislative hearings and regulatory comment periods
- mobilizing constituents to contact representatives and participate in advocacy campaigns
- partnering with advocacy organizations amplifying impact
- using media including op-eds, letters to editors, and social media to raise awareness
- supporting or opposing specific legislation through endorsements and grassroots organizing
- participating in comment periods for regulatory changes
- voting and encouraging civic participation
- running for office or supporting social work candidates

NASW and state chapters provide policy advocacy infrastructure, toolkits, and alerts enabling member participation. Policy advocacy represents professional responsibility, not optional activity. Social workers possess expertise and credibility on health equity, social determinants, and vulnerable populations that legislators need for informed decision-making.

## Critical Thinking Questions

1. Analyze HIPAA privacy regulations through a critical information studies lens examining power, surveillance, and whose interests are served. How might HIPAA balance individual privacy against institutional convenience, law enforcement access, and commercial interests in health data? What alternative privacy frameworks might better protect vulnerable populations, including undocumented immigrants, abuse survivors, and individuals with stigmatized conditions?
2. Evaluate EMTALA's effectiveness in preventing patient dumping and ensuring emergency access. What evidence exists regarding EMTALA's actual impact on access equity across insurance status, race, and geography? How do hospitals navigate EMTALA requirements while managing financial pressures, and what does this reveal about tensions between health care as a market commodity versus a human right? What policy alternatives might better ensure access?

## Key Takeaways

- Legal knowledge strengthens social work practice by enabling advocacy, protecting rights, preventing liability, and revealing where laws perpetuate injustice.
- HIPAA establishes national privacy standards permitting PHI disclosure for treatment, payment, and operations while granting patients rights to access and control information.
- EMTALA requires Medicare-participating hospitals to screen and stabilize anyone presenting for emergency care regardless of payment ability, preventing patient dumping.
- ADA prohibits disability discrimination and requires reasonable accommodations, accessible communication, and program modifications in health care settings.

# Section III References


Acierno, R., Hernandez, M. A., Amstadter, A. B., Resnick, H. S., Steve, K., Muzzy, W., & Kilpatrick, D. G. (2010). Prevalence and correlates of emotional, physical, sexual, and financial abuse and potential neglect in the United States: The National Elder Mistreatment Study. *American Journal of Public Health, 100*(2), 292–297. https://doi.org/10.2105/AJPH.2009.163089

Administration for Children and Families. (2019). *Child abuse and neglect prevention: A guide for states*. U.S. Department of Health and Human Services.

Alvarez, K. M., Donohue, B., Carpenter, A., Romero, V., Allen, D. N., & Cross, C. (2010). Development and preliminary evaluation of a training method to assist professionals in reporting suspected child maltreatment. *Child Maltreatment, 15*(3), 211–218. https://doi.org/10.1177/1077559510365535

Anfang, S. A., & Appelbaum, P. S. (2006). Twenty years after Tarasoff: Reviewing the duty to protect. *Harvard Review of Psychiatry, 14*(2), 67–76. https://doi.org/10.1080/10673220600586459

Appelbaum, P. S. (2007). Clinical practice: Assessment of patients' competence to consent to treatment. *New England Journal of Medicine, 357*(18), 1834–1840. https://doi.org/10.1056/NEJMcp074045

Bailey, Z. D., Krieger, N., Agénor, M., Graves, J., Linos, N., & Bassett, M. T. (2017). Structural racism and health inequities in the USA: Evidence and interventions. *The Lancet, 389*(10077), 1453–1463. https://doi.org/10.1016/S0140-6736(17)30569-X

Baines, D. (Ed.). (2017). *Doing anti-oppressive practice: Social justice social work* (3rd ed.). Fernwood Publishing.

Banerjee, M. M. (2011). Social work scholars' representation of Rawls: A critique. *Journal of Social Work Education, 47*(2), 189–211. https://doi.org/10.5175/JSWE.2011.200900063

Beauchamp, T. L., & Childress, J. F. (2019). *Principles of biomedical ethics* (8th ed.). Oxford University Press.

Braveman, P. (2006). Health disparities and health equity: Concepts and measurement. *Annual Review of Public Health, 27*, 167–194. https://doi.org/10.1146/annurev.publhealth.27.021405.102103

Braveman, P., Egerter, S., & Williams, D. R. (2011). The social determinants of health: Coming of age. *Annual Review of Public Health, 32*, 381–398. https://doi.org/10.1146/annurev-publhealth-031210-101218

Brock, D. W. (2008). Philosophical justifications of informed consent in research. In E. J. Emanuel, C. Grady, R. A. Crouch, R. K. Lie, F. G. Miller, & D. Wendler (Eds.), *The Oxford textbook of clinical research ethics* (pp. 606–612). Oxford University Press.

Charles, C., Gafni, A., & Whelan, T. (1997). Shared decision-making in the medical encounter: What does it mean? (Or it takes at least two to tango). *Social Science & Medicine, 44*(5), 681–692. https://doi.org/10.1016/S0277-9536(96)00221-3

Diez Roux, A. V., & Mair, C. (2010). Neighborhoods and health. *Annals of the New York Academy of Sciences, 1186*, 125–145. https://doi.org/10.1111/j.1749-6632.2009.05333.x

Dolgoff, R., Harrington, D., & Loewenberg, F. M. (2012). *Ethical decisions for social work practice* (9th ed.). Brooks/Cole.

Egyud, A., Stephens, K., Swanson-Biearman, B., DiCuccio, M., & Whiteman, K. (2017). Implementation of human trafficking education and treatment algorithm in the emergency department. *Journal of Emergency Nursing, 43*(6), 526–531. https://doi.org/10.1016/j.jen.2017.01.008

Epstein, E. G., & Delgado, S. (2010). Understanding and addressing moral distress. *Online Journal of Issues in Nursing, 15*(3), Manuscript 1. https://doi.org/10.3912/OJIN.Vol15No03Man01

Faden, R. R., & Beauchamp, T. L. (1986). *A history and theory of informed consent*. Oxford University Press.

Feldman, F. (1978). *Introductory ethics*. Prentice-Hall.

Section IV

# Teamwork and System Navigation

Medical social work requires collaboration within complex systems. Practitioners work with diverse professionals, navigate organizational structures, and coordinate across health care and community settings. Effectiveness depends on communication skills, systems thinking, and relationship building (D'Amour et al., 2005). This section develops competencies for team collaboration and system navigation through five focused chapters addressing communication, care coordination, documentation, resource leverage, and conflict management.

The five chapters in this section build competencies in communication, coordination, documentation, resource navigation, and conflict resolution:

**Chapter 16: Communicating With Interdisciplinary Teams** examines evidence-based communication strategies for working within health care teams, including how social workers articulate the profession's unique contributions, navigate professional hierarchies, and use structured frameworks like SBAR to improve team coordination.

**Chapter 17: Coordinating Care Across Systems** addresses the practical and relational work of linking patients to services across fragmented health care and community systems, examining how social workers manage transitions, negotiate service gaps, and sustain continuity of care.

**Chapter 18: Documentation That Matters** explores how clinical documentation functions as both a professional record and an advocacy tool, covering best practices for psychosocial assessment documentation, interdisciplinary communication, and meeting legal and accreditation standards.

**Chapter 19: Leveraging Community Resources** equips practitioners with strategies for identifying, vetting, and mobilizing community-based services and supports, with attention to resource gaps, eligibility barriers, and relationship building with partner organizations.

**Chapter 20: Navigating Family and Team Conflicts** presents frameworks for understanding and de-escalating conflict in clinical settings, addressing disagreements between family members, between patients and providers, and within interdisciplinary teams.

Together, these chapters equip social workers to function as skilled connectors and collaborators within complex systems, able to communicate with clarity, coordinate with precision, document with purpose, and navigate conflict with confidence.

CHAPTER 16

# Communicating with Interdisciplinary Teams

## Learning Objectives

By the end of this chapter, you will be able to do the following:

- Apply evidence-based communication strategies in health care teams
- Articulate social work's unique contributions
- Navigate professional hierarchies effectively
- Utilize SBAR framework

## The Imperative for Collaboration

Health care complexity requires interprofessional teamwork. Research links effective collaboration with reduced mortality, fewer errors, improved patient satisfaction, and better chronic disease management (Reeves et al., 2017). Social workers contribute biopsychosocial perspective, systems thinking, and resource navigation expertise distinguishing them from other disciplines.

**Understanding team roles:** Physicians lead medical decisions, nurses coordinate bedside care, case managers handle insurance and logistics, therapists assess function, pharmacists manage medications, chaplains address spirituality, and social workers provide psychosocial assessment and advocacy. Role clarity prevents duplication while flexibility addresses patient needs (Bronstein, 2003).

## SBAR Communication

SBAR (situation, background, assessment, recommendation) structures clinical communication efficiently (AHRQ, 2014):

- **Situation:** State the immediate concern concisely.
- **Background:** Provide relevant context and history.
- **Assessment:** Offer clinical judgment about the situation.
- **Recommendation:** Propose specific action or request assistance.

**Example:** "Mr. Chen refuses discharge (Situation). He lives alone, has fallen twice monthly, with early dementia noted (Background). I assess inadequate home safety for independent living (Assessment). I recommend short-term rehab placement while arranging home modifications (Recommendation)."

## Building Credibility

Professional influence requires demonstrated competence, effective communication, reliability, understanding of other roles, and patient-centered focus. Speak concisely using clinical rather than emotional language. Prepare thoroughly for team meetings. Follow through on commitments. Frame contributions in terms of shared patient outcomes (Bronstein, 2003).

Avoid over-explaining, excessive deference to medical authority, unpreparedness, and defensiveness. Navigate hierarchies through strategic timing, evidence-based advocacy, documentation, and appropriate escalation when concerns are dismissed.

## Critical Thinking Questions

1. How do professional hierarchies in health care reflect broader social hierarchies of gender, race, and class? What structural changes would create genuinely egalitarian teams?
2. While SBAR improves efficiency, how might it constrain social work's relational knowledge? What gets lost in structured formats?

## Key Takeaways

- Interprofessional collaboration improves outcomes through mutual respect and shared decision-making.
- SBAR provides structured framework ensuring critical information is conveyed efficiently.
- Credibility develops through competence, communication skills, reliability, and patient-centered focus.
- Navigate hierarchies strategically while maintaining commitment to social work perspective.

CHAPTER 17

# Coordinating Care Across Systems

## Learning Objectives

By the end of this chapter, you will be able to do the following:

- Coordinate seamless transitions between care settings
- Navigate multiple systems effectively
- Prevent gaps compromising patient safety
- Implement evidence-based care coordination strategies

## Why Coordination Matters

Care fragmentation creates risks. Approximately 20% of Medicare patients readmit within 30 days, many due to poor care coordination (Jencks et al., 2009). Effective coordination reduces readmissions, improves patient satisfaction, prevents adverse events, and controls costs. Social workers bridge hospital and community systems, addressing medical needs alongside social determinants affecting successful transitions (Coleman et al., 2006).

## Systems Requiring Coordination

**Post-acute care:** Skilled nursing facilities, inpatient rehabilitation, long-term acute care, and home health require different paperwork, authorization processes, and clinical criteria. Social workers navigate insurance requirements, arrange transfers, and communicate patient needs across settings.

**Community services:** Primary care, specialty clinics, mental health, substance use treatment, social services, housing programs, and legal aid require relationship building, warm handoffs, and follow-up ensuring connections occur.

**Essential coordination skills:** Maintain comprehensive resource knowledge, build relationships facilitating referrals, track multiple moving parts without dropping details, follow through consistently, document coordination activities clearly, and communicate across professional and organizational boundaries (Powell Davies et al., 2008).

## The Warm Handoff

Direct connection between providers strengthens transitions more than simply providing referral lists. Warm handoffs involve speaking by phone or in person, providing social context beyond medical facts, identifying red flags and strengths, confirming patient understanding, and following up verifying connection occurred. This builds trust between systems and reduces patient burden of repeatedly explaining their situation (Coleman et al., 2006).

## Organizational Strategies

Use tracking systems for referrals and follow-ups, develop standardized templates for common referrals, maintain updated contact directories, color-code tasks by urgency or deadline, and schedule dedicated time for coordination activities rather than fitting them between other tasks. Systematic approaches prevent gaps when managing multiple complex cases.

## Critical Thinking Questions

1. Apply organizational theory to analyze care fragmentation. How do institutional boundaries, payment structures, and professional silos create coordination failures? What would integrated systems require?
2. Examine care coordination as potential burden on patients and families. How might coordination efforts inadvertently increase complexity patients must navigate? What approaches center patient priorities rather than system convenience?

## Key Takeaways

- Care coordination reduces readmissions and improves outcomes by ensuring continuity across settings.
- Multiple systems require navigation including post-acute care, primary care, behavioral health, and community services.
- Warm handoffs build trust between systems and reduce patient burden through direct provider communication.
- Systematic organization prevents gaps when managing multiple complex cases simultaneously.

CHAPTER 18

# Documentation that Matters

## Learning Objectives

By the end of this chapter, you will be able to do the following:

- Document clinically and legally sound notes
- Demonstrate social work value through documentation
- Utilize SOAP and DAP formats appropriately
- Balance thoroughness with efficiency

## Why Documentation Matters

Documentation serves multiple purposes: communicating with team members, establishing need for social work services, creating legal record, supporting continuity across providers, and demonstrating value for reimbursement. Strong documentation protects patients, practitioners, and the profession, while weak documentation creates liability and undermines social work's contributions (Reamer, 2005).

## What to Document

Include psychosocial assessment findings, safety concerns, emotional and mental status observations, social support and family dynamics, functional abilities and limitations, barriers to care and discharge, referrals made and coordination efforts, patient and family education provided, and intervention outcomes. Document facts and observations rather than judgments. Use quotes sparingly but powerfully to capture patient voice (NASW, 2016).

## Documentation Formats

**SOAP:** Subjective (what patient/family reports), Objective (your observations and data), Assessment (clinical interpretation), Plan (interventions and next steps)

**DAP:** Data (combined subjective/objective), Assessment (clinical judgment), Plan (actions and follow-up)

Both formats organize information systematically. Choose the format required by your setting or preferred for the situation. Regardless of format, be specific ("Patient tearful when discussing diagnosis; reports difficulty sleeping, decreased appetite"), avoid jargon, link psychosocial factors to medical care, document delays and barriers for accountability, and write assuming patients will read their records (Reamer, 2005).

## Electronic Health Records

EHRs enable information sharing but create challenges including time burden from templates and required fields, lack of social work-specific functionality, copy-paste errors creating inaccurate records, and reduced narrative quality. Use templates efficiently without sacrificing individualization. Avoid copying forward without verification. Include narrative capturing nuances templates miss.

## What to Avoid

Do not document irrelevant personal details, use vague or judgmental language ("noncompliant" without explanation), include personal opinions unrelated to care, diagnose outside your scope, or document excessively creating burden without added value. Remember that documentation becomes legal record accessible through subpoenas and potentially scrutinized years later. Write professionally and factually.

## Critical Thinking Questions

1. Critique how documentation requirements reflect priorities of health care systems. Whose needs do documentation standards primarily serve: patients, providers, insurers, or institutions?
2. Examine EHR impact on social work practice. How do technological systems shape what gets documented and what remains invisible? What aspects of social work resist standardization?

## Key Takeaways

- Documentation communicates value, creates legal record, supports reimbursement, and ensures continuity.
- SOAP and DAP formats organize information systematically while maintaining clinical focus.
- Strong documentation is specific, avoids jargon, links psychosocial factors to care, and documents barriers.
- EHRs enable sharing but create efficiency and quality challenges requiring intentional management.

CHAPTER 19

# Leveraging Community Resources

## Learning Objectives

By the end of this chapter, you will be able to do the following:

- Identify and access community resources systematically
- Build sustainable resource networks
- Address resource scarcity creatively
- Make effective referrals ensuring follow-through

## The Critical Role of Resource Navigation

Social workers connect patients to resources addressing social determinants of health. Research demonstrates that addressing food insecurity, housing instability, and other social needs improves health outcomes and reduces health care utilization (Garg et al., 2015). Resource navigation requires comprehensive knowledge, relationship building, and systems thinking recognizing that resource access involves more than information provision.

## Types of Community Resources

1. **Basic needs:** Food banks, SNAP enrollment, Meals on Wheels, emergency financial assistance, utility programs, and clothing closets address immediate survival needs.
2. **Housing:** Shelters, transitional housing, permanent supportive housing, housing vouchers, and housing case managers assist unstably housed individuals.
3. **Health care:** Federally qualified health centers, free clinics, medication assistance programs, and Ryan White HIV/AIDS services provide care for uninsured and underinsured populations.
4. **Behavioral health:** Outpatient therapy, support groups, substance use treatment, crisis services, and peer support address mental health and addiction needs.
5. **Legal services:** Legal aid, domestic violence advocates, guardianship assistance, and benefits counseling help navigate legal systems and secure entitlements (Sokol & Fisher, 2016).

## Building Your Resource Toolbox

Maintain organized, updated resource lists. Verify resources personally by calling numbers and visiting locations. Build relationships with community partners facilitating referrals. Understand eligibility requirements preventing inappropriate referrals. Track patient feedback about resource quality. Update information quarterly as resources change. Consider geography, transportation, language, cultural appropriateness, and accessibility when matching resources to patients.

## When Resources Are Scarce

Inevitable resource limitations require creativity. Network with colleagues discovering lesser-known resources. Advocate for expanded services through policy engagement. Develop partnerships with faith communities, civic organizations, and informal supports. Help patients navigate waitlists through follow-up and advocacy. Document unmet needs systematically to support funding requests. Acknowledge limitations honestly while maintaining hope and persistent effort.

## Effective Referral Practices

Explain the referral purpose clearly. Set realistic expectations about waitlists and processes. Involve patients in decision-making about which resources to pursue. Make warm handoffs when possible through joint calls or emails. Provide written information including contact details and directions. Follow up verifying connection occurred. Address barriers preventing follow-through including transportation, phone access, language, and competing priorities. Document referrals made and outcomes for continuity and accountability.

## Critical Thinking Questions

1. Analyze resource scarcity through political economy lens. How do policy choices create resource inadequacy? What would adequately funded safety nets require, and what prevents their development?
2. Examine social workers' role in resource navigation. Does helping individuals access scarce resources inadvertently legitimize inadequate systems? How can individual service provision combine with advocacy for structural change?

## Key Takeaways

- Resource navigation addresses social determinants improving health outcomes and reducing utilization.
- Community resources span basic needs, housing, health care, behavioral health, and legal services.
- Building comprehensive resource knowledge requires verification, relationship-building, and regular updating.
- Effective referrals involve explanation, realistic expectations, patient involvement, warm handoffs, and follow-up.
- Resource scarcity requires creativity, advocacy, documentation of gaps, and honest acknowledgment of limitations.

CHAPTER 20

# Navigating Family and Team Conflicts

## Learning Objectives

By the end of this chapter, you will be able to do the following:

- Facilitate difficult conversations using evidence-based strategies
- Mediate family and team conflicts effectively
- Maintain therapeutic presence during escalation
- Apply conflict resolution frameworks

## Understanding Conflict in Health Care

Conflict emerges when values, goals, or interests collide. Health care generates conflicts around end-of-life decisions, treatment approaches, resource allocation, role boundaries, and communication breakdowns. Conflict itself is not failure but a signal that something important is at stake. Social workers help stakeholders move toward resolution with clarity and respect (Fisher & Ury, 1981).

## Common Conflict Scenarios

**Family disagreements:** Siblings disagree about continuing life support. Surrogates make decisions that others question. Cultural differences create tension about appropriate care. Each person's perspective reflects love and concern expressed differently.

**Team conflicts:** Physicians and nurses disagree about discharge readiness. Disciplines dispute role boundaries. Team members hold different values about quality of life versus life prolongation.

**Patient–provider conflicts:** Patients refuse recommended treatment. Families demand aggressive care clinicians view as futile. Trust breaks down from perceived dismissiveness or discrimination.

## Facilitation Strategies

1. **Set ground rules:** Establish respectful communication norms. Request turn-taking without interruption. Emphasize the shared goal of patient wellbeing despite different perspectives.
2. **Use reflective listening:** Paraphrase to verify understanding: "What I hear you saying is...." Acknowledge emotions without judgment: "This is incredibly difficult, and everyone here cares deeply."

3. **Refocus on patient:** Redirect to patient's known wishes, values, and best interests: "What would your mother want if she could tell us?" Center decision-making on the patient rather than family preferences or professional opinions.
4. **Identify common ground:** Highlight shared goals and values even when proposed solutions differ. Build from agreement toward resolution.
5. **Separate positions from interests:** Explore underlying needs and concerns beneath stated positions. Often apparent conflicts mask compatible underlying interests (Fisher & Ury, 1981).
6. **Know when to escalate:** Some conflicts require an ethics consultation, mediation by supervisors, or legal clarification. Recognize limits and utilize appropriate resources.

## Maintaining Boundaries During Conflict

Conflict activates stress responses. Practice emotional regulation through breathing, grounding, and self-awareness. Avoid taking sides prematurely or personalizing attacks. Maintain therapeutic neutrality while clarifying relevant facts and options. Document conflicts and facilitation efforts thoroughly. Debrief with colleagues after intense situations preventing vicarious traumatization and processing emotions.

## Critical Thinking Questions

1. Analyze conflict through systems theory. How do conflicts often reflect systemic dysfunction rather than individual pathology? When should responses address system-level problems versus interpersonal dynamics?
2. Examine power dynamics in health care conflicts. Whose voices get heard and whose get marginalized? How can social workers facilitate processes that genuinely equalize power rather than reinforcing existing hierarchies?

## Key Takeaways

- Conflict signals important issues at stake and creates opportunities for clarification and resolution.
- Common conflicts involve family disagreements, team disputes, and patient–provider tensions around values and decisions.
- Effective facilitation uses ground rules, reflective listening, patient-centered refocusing, and interest exploration.
- Emotional regulation and clear boundaries enable social workers to remain therapeutic during escalation.
- Know when to escalate to ethics consultation, mediation, or legal clarification beyond frontline facilitation.

# Section IV References


Agency for Healthcare Research and Quality. (2014). *TeamSTEPPS 2.0*. https://www.ahrq.gov/teamstepps/index.html

Bronstein, L. R. (2003). A model for interdisciplinary collaboration. *Social Work, 48*(3), 297–306. https://doi.org/10.1093/sw/48.3.297

Coleman, E. A., Parry, C., Chalmers, S., & Min, S. J. (2006). The care transitions intervention: Results of a randomized controlled trial. *Archives of Internal Medicine, 166*(17), 1822–1828. https://doi.org/10.1001/archinte.166.17.1822

D'Amour, D., Ferrada-Videla, M., San Martin Rodriguez, L., & Beaulieu, M. D. (2005). The conceptual basis for interprofessional collaboration. *Journal of Interprofessional Care, 19*(Supplement 1), 116–131. https://doi.org/10.1080/13561820500082529

Fisher, R., & Ury, W. (1981). *Getting to yes: Negotiating agreement without giving in*. Penguin Books.

Garg, A., Toy, S., Tripodis, Y., Silverstein, M., & Freeman, E. (2015). Addressing social determinants of health at well child care visits. *Pediatrics, 135*(2), e296–e304. https://doi.org/10.1542/peds.2014-2367

Jencks, S. F., Williams, M. V., & Coleman, E. A. (2009). Rehospitalizations among patients in the Medicare fee-for-service program. *New England Journal of Medicine, 360*(14), 1418–1428. https://doi.org/10.1056/NEJMsa0803563

National Association of Social Workers. (2016). *NASW standards for social work practice in health care settings*. NASW Press.

Powell Davies, G., Williams, A. M., Larsen, K., Perkins, D., Roland, M., & Harris, M. F. (2008). Coordinating primary health care. *Medical Journal of Australia, 188*(Supplement 8), S65–S68. https://doi.org/10.5694/j.1326-5377.2008.tb01748.x

Reamer, F. G. (2005). Documentation in social work: Evolving ethical and risk-management standards. *Social Work, 50*(4), 325–334. https://doi.org/10.1093/sw/50.4.325

Reeves, S., Pelone, F., Harrison, R., Goldman, J., & Zwarenstein, M. (2017). Interprofessional collaboration to improve professional practice and healthcare outcomes. *Cochrane Database of Systematic Reviews, 6*, CD000072. https://doi.org/10.1002/14651858.CD000072.pub3

Sokol, R., & Fisher, E. (2016). Peer support for the hardly reached. *American Journal of Public Health, 106*(7), 1209–1211. https://doi.org/10.2105/AJPH.2016.303180

Section V

# Growth and Leadership in Social Work

Medical social work demands continuous growth. The field evolves, health care systems change, research generates new knowledge, and practitioners develop across career spans. Sustainable, effective practice requires attending to professional development, maintaining well-being, and cultivating leadership regardless of formal position. This section addresses personal and professional growth through five chapters examining self-care, licensure and supervision, cultural humility, mentorship, and staying current in a changing field.

The five chapters in this section support practitioners in building sustainable, evolving, and leadership-oriented careers:

**Chapter 21: Building a Self-Care Practice** addresses the realities of burnout, compassion fatigue, and vicarious trauma in medical social work, offering evidence-based strategies for sustainable self-care and work–life integration that protect both practitioner wellbeing and patient care quality.

**Chapter 22: Licensure, Supervision, and Career Development** maps the professional development landscape for social workers in health care settings, covering licensure pathways, the supervisory relationship, continuing education, and intentional career planning across career stages.

**Chapter 23: Practicing Cultural Humility** moves beyond static competence models to examine cultural humility as a lifelong practice, exploring how ongoing self-reflection, power analysis, and relationship-centered engagement enable more equitable, responsive care.

**Chapter 24: Mentorship and Teaching in the Medical Setting** examines the responsibilities of experienced practitioners to support the next generation, covering formal and informal mentorship, clinical supervision, student field education, and creating learning environments in health care settings.

**Chapter 25: Staying Current in a Changing Field** explores strategies for engaging with emerging research, evolving policy, and shifting practice standards, positioning social workers as active contributors to the knowledge base rather than passive consumers.

These chapters affirm that professional growth is not incidental to effective practice—it is integral to it. The social worker who invests in self-care, cultural learning, mentorship, and ongoing knowledge development brings a fuller, more resilient, and more effective presence to every patient encounter.

CHAPTER 21

# Building a Self-Care Practice

## Learning Objectives

By the end of this chapter, you will be able to do the following:

- Recognize signs of burnout and compassion fatigue
- Implement evidence-based self-care strategies
- Establish sustainable work-life integration
- Access organizational support systems

## The Reality of Burnout

Medical social work creates risk for burnout, compassion fatigue, and vicarious trauma. Burnout involves emotional exhaustion, depersonalization, and a reduced sense of accomplishment resulting from chronic workplace stress (Maslach & Leiter, 2016). Compassion fatigue emerges from absorbing others' suffering, creating symptoms resembling PTSD, including intrusive thoughts, emotional numbing, and hyperarousal (Figley, 1995). Research documents high burnout rates among health care social workers, with consequences including decreased job satisfaction, intention to leave the profession, reduced quality of care, and physical health problems (Lloyd et al., 2002).

### Recognizing Warning Signs

Burnout manifests as dreading work, feeling emotionally drained after interactions, cynicism about patients or the profession, reduced empathy, difficulty concentrating, physical symptoms (headaches, gastrointestinal issues, sleep disturbance), and withdrawal from colleagues. Early recognition enables intervention before complete depletion occurs.

## Evidence-Based Self-Care Strategies

Self-care is not selfish but essential for sustainable practice. Research identifies effective approaches across multiple domains (Lee & Miller, 2013):

1. **Physical self-care:** Regular exercise, adequate sleep, nutritious eating, and medical care form the foundation. Physical health directly affects stress resilience and emotional capacity.
2. **Emotional self-care:** Therapy, journaling, creative expression, and emotional processing with trusted others prevent accumulation of unprocessed feelings. Normalize seeking mental health support as professional strength rather than weakness.
3. **Professional self-care:** Clear boundaries between work and personal life, realistic caseload man-

agement, regular supervision, continuing education maintaining engagement, and saying no to excessive demands protect against overextension.

4. **Relational self-care:** Meaningful time with loved ones, social connection beyond work, and relationships where you receive rather than always give replenish emotional resources.
5. **Spiritual self-care:** Activities connecting with meaning and purpose, including meditation, religious practice, philosophical reflection, or immersing oneself in nature, sustain a sense of calling that brought you to social work.

## Workplace Micro-Practices

Brief practices integrated into workdays provide immediate stress reduction. Between patient encounters, practice 4-7-8 breathing (inhale 4 counts, hold 7, exhale 8). Step outside for two minutes of fresh air or sunlight. Listen to calming music during documentation. Use grounding objects or scents. Take actual lunch breaks away from your workspace. These small practices accumulate to significant stress reduction (Sanchez-Reilly et al., 2013).

## Setting Boundaries

Burnout often results from saying yes to everything. Boundaries are ethical practice, not selfishness. Leave work on time when possible. Don't check work email after hours unless explicitly required. Protect breaks and mealtimes. Decline additional responsibilities when already at capacity. Communicate limits clearly and unapologetically. Boundaries model healthy practice and prevent resentment eroding care quality.

## Organizational Responsibility

While individual self-care matters, organizations bear responsibility for creating sustainable work environments. Advocate for reasonable caseloads, adequate supervision, debriefing after traumatic events, institutional support for continuing education, and cultures valuing practitioner wellness. When organizations systematically understaff, demand excessive productivity, or ignore moral distress, individual self-care proves insufficient. Collective advocacy and, sometimes, leaving toxic environments become necessary.

## Critical Thinking Questions

1. Critique how self-care discourse places responsibility on individuals rather than addressing organizational and systemic factors creating unsustainable work conditions. What structural changes would make health care work genuinely sustainable?
2. Examine privilege dimensions of self-care advice. How do recommendations assume resources (e.g., time, money, childcare) that are not equally available? What would equity-informed self-care acknowledge?

## Key Takeaways

- Burnout and compassion fatigue represent occupational hazards requiring recognition and active management.
- Evidence-based self-care spans physical, emotional, professional, relational, and spiritual domains.

- Workplace micro-practices and clear boundaries provide immediate stress reduction.
- Organizations bear responsibility for sustainable work conditions beyond individual self-care.

CHAPTER 22

# Licensure, Supervision, and Career Development

## Learning Objectives

By the end of this chapter, you will be able to do the following:

- Understand licensure requirements and career implications
- Utilize clinical supervision effectively for growth
- Plan intentional career trajectories
- Pursue continuing education strategically

## Social Work Licensure

Licensure regulates social work practice, ensuring minimum competency standards while defining scope of practice. Requirements vary by state but typically include tiered levels (Barker & Branson, 2014):

**LMSW/LGSW (licensed master/graduate social worker):** Entry-level license requiring MSW degree, passing the master's level licensing exam, and often supervised practice hours. Permits practice under supervision but not independent clinical practice or diagnosis.

**LCSW (licensed clinical social worker):** Advanced license requiring additional supervised clinical hours (typically 3,000 hours over 2 years), passing clinical exam, and demonstrated competence. Permits independent practice, clinical assessment, and psychotherapy.

**Specialized credentials:** Some states offer additional designations. National certifications include C-ASWCM (advanced social work case manager), ACHP-SW (advanced certified hospice and palliative social worker), and others.

Know your state's specific requirements including supervision hour requirements, continuing education mandates, renewal timelines, and practice restrictions at each license level. Track hours, CEUs, and renewal dates, systematically preventing lapses.

## Clinical Supervision as Growth Opportunity

Supervision provides space for reflection, skill development, ethical reasoning, and emotional processing. Effective supervision explores challenging cases, addresses skill gaps, supports ethical decision-making, processes emotional responses to difficult work, encourages critical thinking, and facilitates career development (Kadushin & Harkness, 2014).

**Maximizing supervision:** Come prepared with specific cases or questions. Reflect on emotional reactions, not just logistics. Request feedback on areas for growth. Discuss professional identity development. Ask to explore theoretical frameworks applying to your practice. Use supervision for genuine learning rather than merely reporting activities.

**When supervision is inadequate:** If supervision proves unhelpful, discuss concerns directly with your supervisor. Request different approaches or focus areas. Seek additional supervision or consultation from colleagues. Consider external supervision if institutional supervision remains insufficient. Quality supervision is a professional right, not a luxury.

## Intentional Career Development

Career paths in medical social work vary widely. Advancement might involve moving into leadership or program development, specializing in particular populations or conditions (oncology, transplant, palliative care), supervising students and new professionals, transitioning to education or research, developing private practice, engaging in policy advocacy, or combining clinical work with consultation or training.

Rather than defaulting to whatever opportunities arise, develop intentional career vision. Reflect on what energizes you, what skills you want to develop, what impact you seek, what work-life balance you need, and what aligns with your values. Seek mentors doing work you admire. Say yes to opportunities stretching your abilities. Invest in professional development advancing your goals.

## Continuing Education Strategy

Beyond meeting license requirements, continuing education maintains competence in evolving field. Choose education genuinely interesting and relevant rather than merely convenient or cheap. Attend conferences providing networking alongside learning. Pursue certifications demonstrating specialized expertise. Read professional journals regularly. Engage with professional organizations. Learning represents career-long commitment, not finite achievement.

## Critical Thinking Questions

1. Analyze licensure as professional gatekeeping. While ensuring minimum standards, how might licensure create barriers to entry that disproportionately affect marginalized communities? What would more equitable credentialing look like?
2. Examine career development through the lens of social location. How do race, class, gender, disability, and other identities shape career trajectories and advancement opportunities in social work?

## Key Takeaways

- Licensure requirements vary by state but typically include tiered levels from master's to clinical licenses.
- Clinical supervision provides essential space for reflection, skill development, and emotional processing.
- Intentional career development involves reflecting on values, seeking mentors, and pursuing opportunities aligned with goals.

- Continuing education maintains competence and engagement beyond minimum license requirements
- Track supervision hours, CEUs, and renewal dates systematically to prevent licensure lapses.

CHAPTER 23

# Practicing Cultural Humility

## Learning Objectives

By the end of this chapter, you will be able to do the following:

- Apply cultural humility as ongoing practice rather than achieved competence
- Examine personal biases and assumptions continuously
- Engage in lifelong cultural learning
- Center marginalized voices and knowledge

## Cultural Humility as Lifelong Commitment

Cultural competence frameworks suggest achievable mastery of cultural knowledge. Cultural humility instead emphasizes lifelong learning, critical self-reflection, and recognition that complete understanding of cultures other than one's own remains impossible (Tervalon & Murray-García, 1998). This shift proves essential because competence language implies endpoint while humility acknowledges ongoing process requiring continuous growth, discomfort, and change.

### Three Core Commitments

1. **Lifelong learning:** Actively seek understanding through reading, training, community engagement, and learning from patients. Recognize that cultural knowledge continually evolves. Remain open to correction and new understanding. Approach each patient as unique individual rather than representative of cultural group.
2. **Critical self-reflection:** Examine your own cultural identity, values, assumptions, privileges, and biases regularly. Consider how your background shapes clinical perceptions and interactions. Notice when discomfort arises in cross-cultural encounters and explore its sources. Acknowledge complicity in oppressive systems even with good intentions.
3. **Power-sharing:** Recognize power differentials in professional relationships and work actively to minimize them. Honor patient expertise about their own lives. Support patient-centered care and shared decision-making. Advocate for organizational changes addressing systemic inequities (Hook et al., 2013).

## Examining Implicit Bias

Implicit biases operate unconsciously, affecting judgments despite explicit commitments to equality. Health care providers, including social workers, harbor biases affecting pain management, diagnostic accuracy, treatment recommendations, and communication quality. Taking Implicit Association Tests (implicit.harvard.edu) reveals unconscious biases as starting point for change.

**Addressing bias:** Increase awareness through assessment and reflection. Slow down decision-making when stakes are high, as bias increases under time pressure. Use structured tools and check-lists reducing intuitive judgment's influence. Seek diverse perspectives through consultation. Build meaningful relationships with diverse communities. Hold yourself accountable through supervision and peer review (Burgess et al., 2017).

## Centering Marginalized Voices

Cultural humility requires centering rather than speaking for marginalized communities. This means following leadership of affected communities in advocacy work, seeking out and amplifying marginalized voices in research and policy, paying for consultation from community experts, deferring to lived experience as expertise, and examining when professional perspectives dismiss or override community knowledge. Humility involves recognizing what you don't know and who knows better.

## Ongoing Cultural Learning

Cultural humility demands continuous learning through diverse reading beyond mainstream social work literature, attending trainings challenging rather than confirming existing perspectives, engaging with communities different from your own, learning from patients about their cultural experiences, staying current with social justice movements, and reflecting regularly on growth areas and blind spots.

## Critical Thinking Questions

1. Analyze how cultural humility frameworks might still center professional perspectives and power. What would genuinely decolonized practice look like, and what might it require practitioners to relinquish?
2. Examine the limits of individual cultural humility when working within structurally oppressive systems. How can practitioners practice humility while institutions remain culturally violent?

## Key Takeaways

- Cultural humility emphasizes lifelong learning and critical self-reflection rather than achieved competence.
- Three core commitments include continuous learning, examining personal biases and power, and sharing power.
- Ongoing learning requires diverse reading, challenging training, community engagement, and regular reflection.
- Implicit bias affects clinical judgments despite explicit equality commitments, requiring active management.
- Centering marginalized voices means following community leadership and deferring to lived experience.

CHAPTER 24

# Mentorship and Teaching in the Medical Setting

## Learning Objectives

By the end of this chapter, you will be able to do the following:

- Engage in effective mentorship practices
- Supervise social work students and interns competently
- Lead through example and education
- Develop sustainable mentorship relationships

## Why Mentorship Matters

Medical social work's demands create steep learning curves and high turnover. Mentorship provides support, skill development, professional socialization, and retention improvement. Research links quality mentorship with increased job satisfaction, reduced burnout, improved clinical skills, and career advancement (Mor Barak et al., 2009). Mentorship benefits mentors through renewed purpose, perspective from fresh eyes, skill development in teaching and supervision, and satisfaction from contributing to the profession's future.

## Forms of Leadership

You need not hold formal leadership titles to lead. Leadership emerges through informal mentorship offering guidance to newer colleagues, field instruction supervising MSW students, teaching contributions through presentations or training, advocacy modeling demonstrating ethical practice, and supportive presence for overwhelmed teammates. Every interaction provides opportunities to lead through integrity and competence.

## Effective Mentorship Practices

1. **Create psychological safety:** Make it okay to not know, struggle, or make mistakes. Share your own challenges and learning experiences. Respond to questions without judgment. Normalize stress and uncertainty inherent in the work.
2. **Provide concrete guidance:** Balance emotional support with practical skill-building. Model techniques, review documentation, practice difficult conversations, and provide specific feedback on strengths and growth areas.

3. **Encourage reflection:** Ask "What felt most challenging?"
   "What surprised you?"
   "What would you do differently?"
   Guide critical thinking rather than simply provide answers.
4. **Be available and reliable:** Honor commitments. Make time for regular check-ins. Respond to questions promptly. Demonstrate that you value the relationship.
5. **Set appropriate boundaries:** Mentorship involves guidance, not friendship or therapy. Maintain professional boundaries while being warm and supportive. End formal mentoring relationships when appropriate, transitioning to collegial relationships (Bogo, 2015).

## Supervising Students

Field instruction shapes future social workers. Effective student supervision involves clear expectations and learning objectives, regular supervision meetings with protected time, progressive skill-building appropriate to student level, constructive feedback balancing affirmation with growth challenges, cultural responsiveness and anti-oppressive supervision, and evaluation processes that are fair and developmental. Students remember supervisors who believed in them, challenged them appropriately, and modeled the profession's values.

## Critical Thinking Questions

1. Analyze mentorship through a lens of professional reproduction. How do mentoring relationships risk reproducing existing professional norms and power structures? How might mentorship support transformative rather than reproductive professional development?
2. Examine who receives mentorship and who becomes a mentor. What patterns of privilege and marginalization affect mentoring access and quality? How can mentorship address rather than perpetuate inequities?

## Key Takeaways

- Mentorship improves job satisfaction, reduces burnout, develops skills, and supports retention.
- Leadership occurs through informal mentorship, student supervision, teaching, advocacy, and supportive presence.
- Effective practices include creating safety, providing concrete guidance, encouraging reflection, and maintaining boundaries.
- Field instruction shapes future social workers through clear expectations, regular supervision, and developmental feedback.
- Examine how mentorship might reproduce or challenge existing professional norms and power structures.

CHAPTER 25

# Staying Current in a Changing Field

## Learning Objectives

By the end of this chapter, you will be able to do the following:

- Engage in evidence-based practice through ongoing learning
- Maintain awareness of health care trends and policy changes
- Contribute to practice-based evidence
- Participate in professional communities

## The Imperative for Lifelong Learning

Health care evolves continuously. New research emerges, policies change, technologies advance, and populations' needs shift. Remaining effective requires ongoing learning beyond initial education and licensure. Evidence-based practice integrates best available research with clinical expertise and patient values to guide decisions (Rubin & Parrish, 2012). This demands staying current with research, critically evaluating evidence, and adapting practice based on new knowledge.

## What to Follow

1. **Health care policy:** Changes in insurance coverage, Medicaid policy, Medicare regulations, and health care law affect patient access and social work practice. Follow CMS updates, NASW policy alerts, and health care policy news affecting your practice area.
2. **Medical advances:** New treatments, diagnostic tools, and disease understanding affect care planning. You need not master medical details but should understand basics of treatments your patients receive and how they affect quality of life and functioning.
3. **Social work research:** Professional journals including *Health & Social Work*, *Social Work in Health Care*, and *Journal of Social Work in End-of-Life & Palliative Care* publish relevant research. Read journals in your specialty area regularly.
4. **Social determinants and health equity:** Research on structural racism, social determinants, and health disparities evolves rapidly. Stay current with equity scholarship informing advocacy and practice.
5. **Best practices:** Evidence-based intervention models, assessment tools, and practice guidelines develop continuously. Follow specialty organizations for practice updates in your area (Holden et al., 2012).

## Strategies for Staying Informed

1. **Dedicate time for reading:** Schedule regular time for professional reading rather than squeezing it in sporadically. Even 30 minutes weekly accumulates substantial learning.
2. **Join professional organizations:** NASW, specialty organizations (Society for Social Work Leadership in Health Care, NASW specialty practice sections), and interdisciplinary groups provide education, networking, and updates.
3. **Attend conferences:** Annual conferences offer intensive learning, networking, and exposure to emerging issues. Virtual options increase accessibility.
4. **Participate in communities of practice:** Journal clubs, peer consultation groups, and online communities facilitate learning and support. Learning occurs through dialogue, not isolation.
5. **Contribute to knowledge:** Share practice wisdom through presentations, publications, or informal teaching. Articulating knowledge strengthens understanding and contributes to professional knowledge base.

## Practice-Based Evidence

Evidence-based practice flows from research to practice, but practice-based evidence reverses the flow, systematically documenting what works in real-world practice to inform research and theory (Epstein, 2011). Social workers contribute by documenting outcomes systematically, sharing successful innovations, participating in practice-based research, and challenging research that doesn't reflect practice realities.

## Critical Thinking Questions

1. Critique evidence-based practice paradigms. What forms of knowledge do they privilege and marginalize? How might emphasis on quantitative research devalue practice wisdom, client voice, and community knowledge?
2. Examine who produces knowledge deemed credible in social work. How do academic-practice hierarchies affect what counts as evidence? What would democratized knowledge production look like?

## Key Takeaways

- Lifelong learning maintains competence as health care, policy, and research evolve continuously.
- Follow health care policy, medical advances, social work research, health equity scholarship, and best practices.
- Strategies include dedicated reading time, involvement in professional organizations, conference attendance, and participation in communities of practice.
- Practice-based evidence documents what works in real-world settings, complementing research-to-practice flow.
- Critically examine what forms of knowledge are privileged in evidence hierarchies and whose voices are marginalized.

# Section V References


Barker, R. L., & Branson, D. M. (2014). *Forensic social work: Legal aspects of professional practice* (3rd ed.). Routledge.

Bogo, M. (2015). *Field education for professional expertise: Integrating field and classroom learning*. Columbia University Press.

Burgess, D. J., Beach, M. C., & Saha, S. (2017). Mindfulness practice: A promising approach to reducing the effects of clinician implicit bias on patients. *Patient Education and Counseling, 100*(2), 372–376. https://doi.org/10.1016/j.pec.2016.09.005

Epstein, I. (2011). Reconciling evidence-based practice, evidence-informed practice, and practice-based research. *Social Work, 56*(3), 284–288. https://doi.org/10.1093/sw/56.3.284

Figley, C. R. (Ed.). (1995). *Compassion fatigue: Coping with secondary traumatic stress disorder in those who treat the traumatized*. Brunner/Mazel.

Holden, G., Barker, K., Meenaghan, T., & Rosenberg, G. (2012). Professional development: A study of the health care and social assistance sector. *Journal of Evidence-Based Social Work, 9*(1–2), 183–209. https://doi.org/10.1080/15433714.2012.633235

Hook, J. N., Davis, D. E., Owen, J., Worthington, E. L., & Utsey, S. O. (2013). Cultural humility: Measuring openness to culturally diverse clients. *Journal of Counseling Psychology, 60*(3), 353–366. https://doi.org/10.1037/a0032595

Kadushin, A., & Harkness, D. (2014). *Supervision in social work* (5th ed.). Columbia University Press.

Lee, J. J., & Miller, S. E. (2013). A self-care framework for social workers: Building a strong foundation for practice. *Families in Society, 94*(2), 96–103. https://doi.org/10.1606/1044-3894.4289

Lloyd, C., King, R., & Chenoweth, L. (2002). Social work, stress and burnout: A review. *Journal of Mental Health, 11*(3), 255–265. https://doi.org/10.1080/09638230020023642

Maslach, C., & Leiter, M. P. (2016). Understanding the burnout experience: Recent research and its implications for psychiatry. *World Psychiatry, 15*(2), 103–111. https://doi.org/10.1002/wps.20311

Mor Barak, M. E., Travis, D. J., Pyun, H., & Xie, B. (2009). The impact of supervision on worker outcomes: A meta-analysis. *Social Service Review, 83*(1), 3–32. https://doi.org/10.1086/599028

Rubin, A., & Parrish, D. E. (2012). Outcomes of social work intervention with older adults: A systematic review. *Journal of Evidence-Based Social Work, 9*(1–2), 88–107. https://doi.org/10.1080/15433714.2012.636329

Sanchez-Reilly, S., Morrison, L. J., Carey, E., Bernacki, R., O'Neill, L., Kapo, J., Periyakoil, V. S., & Thomas, J. D. (2013). Caring for oneself to care for others: Physicians and their self-care. *Journal of Supportive Oncology, 11*(2), 75–81. https://doi.org/10.12788/j.suponc.0003

Tervalon, M., & Murray-García, J. (1998). Cultural humility versus cultural competence: A critical distinction in defining physician training outcomes in multicultural education. *Journal of Health Care for the Poor and Underserved, 9*(2), 117–125. https://doi.org/10.1353/hpu.2010.0233

# Conclusion

Medical social work represents far more than a profession. It embodies a calling to stand with vulnerable individuals during their most challenging moments, to challenge unjust systems that perpetuate suffering, and to bring humanity to health care environments increasingly dominated by efficiency metrics and cost containment pressures. Throughout these 25 chapters, we have explored the knowledge, skills, and values essential for competent, compassionate, and justice-oriented practice in medical settings.

This journey began with clinical foundations including medical terminology, health care system navigation, common health conditions, psychosocial assessment, and trauma-informed care. These foundational competencies enable social workers to communicate effectively across disciplines, understand the medical context of patients' lives, conduct thorough biopsychosocial assessments, and provide care that honors the full humanity of those we serve. Mastery of these basics proves necessary but insufficient for truly excellent practice.

We then explored the relational heart of medical social work through chapters addressing crisis intervention, grief and loss, cultural competence, discharge planning, and advance care planning. These dimensions of practice reminded us that while technical competence matters, the capacity to be fully present with suffering, to witness pain without attempting to fix everything, and to honor patient autonomy during crisis represents the essence of social work's contribution to health care. Patients and families remember not our documentation skills or discharge planning efficiency but our ability to see them as whole people amid systems that too often reduce them to diagnoses and bed days.

The ethics, advocacy, and equity section positioned social workers as moral anchors within health care teams. Chapters on protecting patient rights, mandated reporting, ethical decision-making, health equity, and health care law affirmed that ethical practice extends beyond avoiding violations to proactively advancing justice. Social workers serve not merely as system navigators helping individuals adapt to unjust structures but as change agents working to transform systems themselves. This dual role of providing individual support while challenging structural inequities distinguishes social work from disciplines focused exclusively on individual-level interventions.

Teamwork and system navigation competencies addressed the collaborative nature of health care practice. Medical social workers function within complex organizational systems, working alongside diverse professionals and coordinating across multiple settings. Effectiveness requires communication skills that build credibility, documentation that demonstrates value, resource networks that enables comprehensive support, and conflict navigation that maintains therapeutic presence amid tension. These chapters recognize that excellent practice involves both skilled collaboration within teams and critical thinking that identifies when systems themselves require transformation.

Finally, the growth and leadership section acknowledged that sustainable practice demands ongoing attention to professional development and personal well-being. Self-care proves essential not as optional luxury but as professional responsibility enabling continued presence for those we serve. Licensure, supervision, cultural humility, mentorship, and staying current represent commitments extending throughout careers rather than achievements completed during graduate education. Leadership emerges not only through formal positions but through modeling ethical practice, supporting colleagues, and contributing to professional knowledge.

## Integrating Knowledge with Practice Wisdom

This book has put together empirical research, theoretical frameworks, practice guidelines, and real-world examples. Evidence-based practice provides crucial foundation, ensuring interventions rest on solid research demonstrating effectiveness. However, evidence-based practice proves insufficient without practice-based evidence, the systematic documentation and analysis of what works in actual clinical encounters with real patients facing complex circumstances that research studies often exclude.

The most skilled medical social workers integrate research knowledge with practice wisdom accumulated through experience, reflection, and ongoing learning. They recognize that no protocol or guideline can anticipate every situation's unique contours. They draw on theoretical frameworks for guidance while remaining flexible enough to adapt when theories inadequately capture patients' lived realities. They honor both quantitative evidence demonstrating intervention effectiveness and qualitative understanding of meaning, context, and relationship that research struggles to measure.

This integration requires practitioners who read research critically, recognizing its contributions and limitations. Who engage in systematic reflection on their own practice, noticing patterns and learning from both successes and failures. Who participate in professional communities where knowledge is collectively constructed through dialogue rather than passively consumed. Who approach patients with genuine curiosity, recognizing that each person teaches us something that books and journals cannot.

## The Ongoing Journey

If you approached this book seeking definitive answers to medical social work's challenges, you may feel disappointed. While we have provided frameworks, strategies, and evidence-based guidance, health care practice's inherent complexity resists formulaic solutions. Patients present with intersecting physical, psychological, social, and spiritual needs defying simple categorization. Systems contain competing demands and limited resources requiring difficult trade-offs. Ethics involve choosing between imperfect options when values conflict. This messiness reflects not professional failure but human reality.

Embracing uncertainty while maintaining commitment to ongoing learning characterizes professional maturity. The most effective practitioners acknowledge what they do not know, seek consultation when uncertain, and remain humble about the limits of their expertise. They recognize that discomfort signals growth opportunities rather than inadequacy. They understand that complexity cannot be eliminated but can be navigated thoughtfully through reflection, collaboration, and continuous learning.

Your journey as a medical social worker will bring challenges this book cannot anticipate. Health care systems will evolve in ways requiring adaptation. You will encounter clinical situations without clear precedents. You will face ethical dilemmas where every option creates harm. You will work within institutions whose policies conflict with patient needs. You will witness suffering you cannot eliminate and systemic injustices you cannot singlehandedly dismantle.

In these moments, return to core social work values. Remember that your primary responsibility involves promoting clients' well-being while advancing social justice. Recognize the inherent dignity and worth of every person you encounter, regardless of diagnosis, behavior, or social circumstances. Understand that relationships serve as vehicles for change, meaning your capacity for authentic human connection matters as much as technical expertise. Practice with integrity, behaving in a trustworthy manner even when no one is watching. Maintain competence through ongoing learning and humble recognition of scope limitations. These values transcend specific interventions or practice settings, providing a compass when navigation proves difficult.

## A Call to Action

Medical social work needs your voice, passion, and commitment to both clinical excellence and social justice. Health care systems increasingly prioritize efficiency over compassion, profit over patients, and individual responsibility over structural change. Social workers must resist these pressures while working within systems to provide excellent care and advocating outside systems for transformation.

This means practicing competently at individual levels, conducting thorough assessments, providing evidence-based interventions, coordinating care effectively, and documenting clearly. It also means recognizing when problems presented as individual deficits actually reflect system failures requiring collective response. When patients cannot afford medications, the problem involves pharmaceutical pricing and insurance coverage, not patient noncompliance. When families struggle to access mental health services, the problem involves inadequate community resources and systemic barriers, not family dysfunction. When patients of color receive inferior care, the problem involves structural racism, not cultural differences.

Effective medical social workers provide excellent individual services while engaging in advocacy, policy work, community organizing, and institutional change efforts addressing root causes of problems they encounter daily. This dual focus proves demanding but essential. Individual interventions without structural advocacy leave systems unchanged, ensuring tomorrow's patients face identical barriers. Structural advocacy without individual competence abandons people suffering now while waiting for future systemic transformation.

You can engage this work at multiple levels. Provide exceptional clinical care reflecting social work values and evidence-based practice. Speak up within institutions when policies or practices harm patients. Participate in professional organizations advancing the profession's knowledge and influence. Engage in policy advocacy supporting health equity and social justice. Build coalitions across disciplines and with community organizations. Support and vote for policies and candidates prioritizing health care access, social determinants, and vulnerable populations. Mentor students and new professionals. Contribute to practice-based evidence through documentation and knowledge sharing. Stay informed and critically engaged with evolving health care landscape.

## Final Reflections

Perhaps the most important lesson from the 25 chapters is this: You are enough. Medical social work's demands can feel overwhelming, creating feelings of inadequacy. You will encounter situations exceeding your current knowledge. You will make mistakes. You will face challenges without clear solutions. This does not mean you are failing. It means you are doing genuine, complex, meaningful work that matters profoundly.

Be patient with yourself as you develop expertise. Seek support from supervisors, colleagues, and mentors. Engage in self-care enabling sustained presence. Practice self-compassion when encountering limitations. Celebrate small victories recognizing that sometimes keeping someone safe for one more day, sitting with grief without offering empty platitudes, or connecting an isolated person to a single resource represents profound success.

Remember why you entered social work. Whether driven by personal experience, passion for justice, desire to help, or sense of calling, reconnect regularly with that motivation. Let it sustain you through difficult moments and remind you that this work matters more than metrics, productivity demands, or institutional pressures suggest.

You will not save everyone. You will not fix broken systems alone. You will not eliminate suffering or solve every problem. What you will do is show up with competence and compassion. You will bear witness to pain. You will advocate for dignity. You will connect people to resources. You will facilitate difficult conversations. You will name injustice. You will support colleagues. You will grow and learn. You will make a difference in ways both visible and invisible.

Medical social work needs you. Patients and families need you. The profession needs you. Health care needs the perspective, values, and skills that only social workers bring. Thank you for your commitment to this essential work. May this book support your journey toward competence, compassion, and enduring clinical impact.

# Appendix A: Case Studies

Applying Knowledge to Practice

The following case studies illustrate key concepts from throughout the book, demonstrating how theoretical frameworks and evidence-based strategies apply in clinical practice. All cases are fictional composites created for educational purposes; any resemblance to actual persons, living or dead, or to real clinical situations is coincidental.

## Case Study 1: The Unsafe Discharge

### Chapter Connections

Chapter 9 (Discharge Planning), Chapter 11 (Patient Rights), Chapter 14 (Health Equity)

### Clinical Scenario

Mr. Rodriguez, a 68-year-old Spanish-speaking man with poorly controlled diabetes, presents to the emergency department with an infected diabetic foot ulcer requiring partial toe amputation. He lives alone in a third-floor walk-up apartment with no elevator. His daughter lives two hours away and works full time. He has Medicaid coverage, limited English proficiency, and no home phone. The medical team plans discharge in three days with home health services.

During psychosocial assessment, you identify multiple safety concerns: inability to safely navigate stairs post-surgery given reduced mobility, lack of family support for wound care and medication management, food insecurity affecting diabetes control, missed medical appointments due to unreliable transportation, and language barriers complicating patient education.

The attending physician states, "We've done all we can medically. He's stable. We need the bed. Home health will handle the rest."

### Analysis Using Chapter Concepts

This situation exemplifies unsafe discharge planning inadequately addressing social determinants of health. Several issues require attention:

*Discharge planning deficits (Chapter 9):* The plan addresses medical stability without assessing psychosocial safety factors. Third-floor walk-up proves unsafe for someone with reduced mobility and a healing foot wound. Home health assumes patient can safely remain home between visits, which this environment does not support. Food insecurity will undermine diabetes management and wound healing.

*Autonomy and safety (Chapter 11):* While Mr. Rodriguez may technically have the capacity to accept discharge, true informed consent requires understanding risks in his language and considering alternatives. Language barriers may prevent genuine informed consent about discharge risks.

*Health equity (Chapter 14):* Multiple social determinants intersect, creating vulnerability: limited English proficiency, Medicaid coverage limiting post-acute options, food insecurity, transportation barriers, and housing inadequacy. Structural factors rather than individual deficits create an unsafe situation.

## Evidence-Based Interventions

1. **Comprehensive SDOH assessment:** Systematically document all social determinants affecting safe discharge including housing accessibility, food security, transportation, social support, language access, and financial resources.
2. **Team advocacy:** Request care conference to present psychosocial barriers to safe discharge. Use SBAR format: "Mr. Rodriguez cannot safely discharge home tomorrow (Situation). He lives in a third-floor walk-up, has active wound requiring care, no caregiver support, food insecurity affecting diabetes, and language barriers (Background). I assess significant fall risk and wound complication risk if discharged as planned (Assessment). I recommend short-term skilled nursing facility placement or intensive home services with environmental modifications (Recommendation)."
3. **Alternative placement exploration:** Investigate skilled nursing facility for short-term rehabilitation and wound care while arranging home modifications (stair lift, first-floor relocation) and increased support services.
4. **Language access:** Ensure professional Spanish interpretation for all medical discussions, discharge teaching, and consent processes. Provide translated materials.
5. **Resource coordination:** Connect to food assistance (SNAP, food bank, Meals on Wheels), arrange Medicaid transportation for follow-up appointments, and explore housing assistance for an accessible unit.
6. **Documentation:** Clearly document all safety concerns, alternatives explored, team discussions, and patient education provided. Note that discharge plan does not adequately address identified risks. This creates record for advocacy and potential appeals if adverse outcomes occur.
7. **Risk management consultation:** If team insists on unsafe discharge despite documented concerns, involve hospital risk management and patient advocacy to escalate appropriately.

## Reflection Questions

1. How do you balance respecting patient autonomy (if Mr. Rodriguez accepts discharge despite risks) with professional responsibility to prevent harm?
2. What systems-level factors create pressure for premature discharge, and how might social workers advocate for structural changes rather than only individual solutions?
3. How do language barriers and Medicaid coverage create different discharge options compared to English-speaking patients with private insurance, and what does this reveal about health inequity?
4. When institutional pressure conflicts with safe discharge planning, what ethical frameworks guide decision-making about escalation versus compromise?

## Key Takeaways

- Safe discharge requires assessing social determinants, not only medical stability.
- Advocacy involves clearly articulating psychosocial risks using evidence and clinical judgment.
- Documentation creates accountability and legal record protecting patients and practitioners.
- Structural inequities including language barriers, insurance coverage, and housing inadequacy create differential discharge safety that social workers must name and address.

# Case Study 2: The Capacity Dilemma

## Chapter Connections

Chapter 11 (Protecting Patient Rights), Chapter 7 (End-of-Life Support), Chapter 13 (Ethical Decision-Making)

## Clinical Scenario

Mrs. Chen, a 79-year-old woman with moderate dementia, is hospitalized with pneumonia. Her daughter (who holds medical power of attorney) insists on signing consent for feeding tube placement, though Mrs. Chen previously completed a living will stating she would not want artificial nutrition if she developed dementia and could not eat independently.

Mrs. Chen appears confused about location and date but recognizes her daughter. When asked about feeding tube, she states, "I want to go home. No tubes." Her daughter responds, "She doesn't understand. She needs this to live. We want everything done."

The medical team seeks social work consultation before proceeding with tube placement.

## Analysis Using Chapter Concepts

This case presents a classic end-of-life ethical dilemma involving capacity questions, advance directive interpretation, surrogate authority, and family dynamics.

*Capacity assessment (Chapter 11):* While Mrs. Chen has dementia, this does not automatically mean she lacks capacity for this specific decision. Formal capacity assessment should evaluate whether she can understand that she has pneumonia affecting swallowing, comprehend that a feeding tube would provide nutrition if she cannot eat, appreciate the consequences of accepting or refusing tube, and communicate a choice. Her statement "no tubes" suggests potential capacity to refuse.

*Advance directive interpretation (Chapter 10):* Mrs. Chen's living will specifically addresses this situation: dementia with inability to eat independently. Her previous clear wishes should guide current decisions unless strong evidence suggests she changed her mind while still having capacity.

*Surrogate authority (Chapter 11):* Medical power of attorney activates when patient lacks capacity. However, surrogates should make substituted judgments based on what patient would want, not what surrogate prefers. Daughter's insistence on "everything" contradicts mother's documented wishes.

*Ethical framework (Chapter 13):* Multiple ethical principles conflict. Autonomy (respecting Mrs. Chen's past and possibly current wishes to refuse), beneficence (feeding tube might prolong life), family wishes (daughter's cultural or emotional needs), and previously stated values (living will refusing artificial nutrition) require careful balancing.

## Evidence-Based Interventions

1. **Formal capacity evaluation:** Request physician or psychologist capacity assessment specifically for feeding tube decision. Use standardized assessment exploring understanding, appreciation, reasoning, and choice expression.
2. **Family meeting:** Facilitate meeting including daughter, medical team, and potentially ethics consultant. Create space for daughter to express fears about mother's death. Explore cultural values about feeding and end-of-life care. Review mother's previously stated wishes.
3. **Clarify advance directive:** Explain that living will specifically addresses this scenario and that daughter's role as surrogate involves honoring mother's wishes, not substituting daughter's preferences.
4. **Explore underlying concerns:** Daughter's insistence may reflect grief, cultural beliefs that stop-

ping feeding equals killing, guilt, or fear. Address these emotions while maintaining focus on patient's preferences.

5. **Palliative care consultation:** Introduce palliative care team to discuss comfort-focused approaches, prognosis with and without feeding tube, and quality versus quantity of life considerations.
6. **Ethics consultation:** If conflict persists, request formal ethics consultation to review case, interview stakeholders, and provide recommendations balancing competing values.
7. **Document thoroughly:** Record capacity evaluation results, advance directive contents, family meeting discussions, patient's statements, and ethical reasoning supporting recommendations.

## Reflection Questions

1. When advance directives conflict with family wishes, how should social workers balance honoring patient's prior autonomous choices with supporting grieving family members?
2. How do cultural values about feeding, family decision-making, and end-of-life care affect interpretation of advance directives created in Western bioethical framework?
3. If capacity evaluation determines Mrs. Chen lacks capacity for this decision, should her current statements ("no tubes") carry any weight against written advance directive and daughter's preferences?
4. What would care ethics versus autonomy-focused ethics suggest about balancing Mrs. Chen's documented wishes, current statements, and daughter's distress?

## Key Takeaways

- Dementia does not equal incapacity; formal assessment of decision-specific capacity is required.
- Surrogate decision-makers should make substituted judgments based on patient's values, not surrogate preferences.
- Advance directives provide crucial guidance but require interpretation when situations arise.
- Family meetings creating space for emotion while maintaining patient-centered focus can facilitate resolution.
- Ethics consultation provides valuable support for complex cases without clear answers.

# Case Study 3: Mandated Reporting Tension

## Chapter Connections

Chapter 12 (Mandated Reporting), Chapter 11 (Patient Rights), Chapter 13 (Ethical Decision-Making)

## Clinical Scenario

Ms. Thompson, a 34-year-old woman, is admitted for treatment of injuries from domestic violence. During psychosocial assessment, she discloses that her partner has hit her multiple times and that she fears for her safety. She has two children, ages 6 and 9, who are not injured but witness the violence.

Ms. Thompson refuses to leave her partner, stating she has nowhere to go and no income, and she fears that he will hurt her worse if she files a police report. She becomes agitated when you mention domestic violence advocacy, stating, "If you tell anyone, he'll know I talked. Please don't report this. I just needed to tell someone."

Your state requires mandatory reporting of domestic violence injuries and child exposure to domestic violence.

## Analysis Using Chapter Concepts

This case presents tension between mandated reporting obligations, patient autonomy, therapeutic relationship, and patient safety.

*Mandated Reporting (Chapter 12):* State law requires reporting domestic violence injuries and child exposure. Failure to report violates legal obligation and could result in professional consequences. However, Ms. Thompson explicitly requests confidentiality and warns that reporting may escalate danger.

*Autonomy (Chapter 11):* Ms. Thompson is a competent adult with the right to make decisions about her safety, including whether to leave her partner or involve authorities. Mandatory reporting removes her control, potentially decreasing future help-seeking.

*Therapeutic Relationship (Chapter 12):* Ms. Thompson trusted you with disclosure. Reporting against her explicit wishes may damage therapeutic alliance and prevent future engagement with services.

*Child Safety (Chapter 12):* Children witnessing domestic violence experience trauma requiring protective intervention. This creates additional reporting obligation separate from adult domestic violence.

## Evidence-Based Interventions

1. **Immediate safety assessment:** Assess lethality risk using validated tool. Explore immediate safety planning including a safe place to go, emergency resources, and signs that danger is escalating.
2. **Transparent communication:** Explain reporting obligations clearly: "I'm required by law to make a report because of your injuries and because your children witness violence. I understand you're afraid of consequences. Let me explain what will happen and how we can try to maximize your safety."
3. **Collaborative reporting:** When possible, involve Ms. Thompson in report process. Explain what will be reported, to whom, and what typically happens next. Offer to make the report together or let her listen to the phone call.
4. **Safety planning:** Work with a domestic violence advocate to develop safety plan addressing immediate and long-term concerns. Identify safe people to contact, important documents to gather, escape routes, and resources available.
5. **Resource connection:** Provide information about domestic violence shelters, legal advocacy, emergency protection orders, financial assistance, and children's trauma services. Respect that she may not be ready to use them now but has information for the future.
6. **Support, not judgment:** Validate her fears and concerns. Explain that leaving abusive relationships is complex process averaging seven attempts before success. Avoid pressuring her to leave if she is not safe or ready.
7. **Child protective services coordination:** When CPS investigates, advocate for services supporting family rather than punitive responses. Emphasize the mother is a protective parent seeking help, not a perpetrator.
8. **Documentation:** Document disclosure, safety assessment, reporting, and resources provided. Note patient's concerns and your clinical reasoning.

## Reflection Questions

1. How do mandatory reporting laws affect power dynamics in therapeutic relationships, particularly for populations already experiencing systemic oppression and surveillance?
2. What does research reveal about domestic violence reporting's actual impact on victim safety, and how should this evidence inform practice when laws require reporting?
3. How can social workers practice trauma-informed care while fulfilling mandated reporting that

removes patient control?

4. What advocacy might address problematic mandatory reporting laws while protecting vulnerable individuals in current legal context?

## Key Takeaways

- Mandated reporting creates genuine ethical tensions between legal obligations, autonomy, and therapeutic relationships.
- Transparency about reporting obligations during informed consent and when disclosures occur maintains trust.
- Collaborative reporting processes involving patients when safe can partially mitigate autonomy loss.
- Safety planning and resource connection provide concrete support alongside mandated reporting.
- Recognize that reporting represents one intervention in a complex situation, not a complete solution.

# Appendix B: Templates and Tools

## Psychosocial Assessment Template

**Patient Information**

- Name, age, date of birth
- Medical record number
- Admission date
- Primary diagnosis/reason for admission
- Anticipated discharge date

**Referral Source and Reason**

- Who requested social work involvement and why

**Mental Health and Emotional Functioning**

- Current mood and affect
- Cognitive status (orientation, memory, attention)
- Coping mechanisms
- History of mental health diagnoses and treatment
- Current psychiatric medications
- Substance use history (current and past)
- Suicidal/homicidal ideation screening

**Social Support System**

- Living situation (with whom, housing type)
- Marital status and relationship quality
- Children and other family members
- Friends and community connections
- Quality and availability of support
- Family dynamics and stressors

**Functional Status**

- Activities of daily living (ADLs): bathing, dressing, toileting, eating, transferring
- Instrumental activities of daily living (IADLs): medication management, meal prep, housekeeping, finances, transportation
- Mobility and ambulation
- Baseline functioning before current illness/injury

**Financial and Insurance**

- Employment status and occupation
- Income sources
- Insurance coverage
- Financial concerns or barriers to care
- Benefit programs (SNAP, SSI/SSDI, etc.)

**Living Environment**

- Housing type and accessibility
- Number of floors, stairs present
- Safety concerns
- Neighborhood resources and safety
- Utilities and housing stability

**Cultural and Spiritual**

- Cultural identity and background
- Primary language
- Health beliefs and practices
- Spiritual or religious affiliation
- Cultural practices important to care

**Legal and Safety**

- Advance directives (living will, medical POA)
- Guardianship or conservatorship
- Legal concerns (custody, court involvement)
- Safety concerns (abuse, domestic violence, exploitation)

**Discharge Planning Needs**

- Anticipated post-acute care needs
- Equipment or home modifications needed
- Services required (home health, rehab, etc.)
- Barriers to safe discharge
- Patient and family goals and preferences

**Strengths and Resources**

- Personal strengths and coping abilities
- Available resources
- Protective factors

**Assessment Summary and Plan**

- Clinical impression
- Priority concerns and needs identified
- Planned interventions and referrals
- Follow-up needed

# Discharge Planning Checklist

☐ **Psychosocial Assessment Completed**

- All relevant domains explored
- Barriers identified
- Strengths documented

☐ **Team Communication**

- Participated in interdisciplinary rounds
- Communicated needs to team members
- Updated on changes in medical status

☐ **Patient and Family Education**

- Diagnosis and treatment explained
- Discharge plan reviewed
- Warning signs identified
- Follow-up appointments scheduled
- Teach-back used to verify understanding

☐ **Post-Acute Care Coordination**

- Level of care determined (home, home health, SNF, rehab, hospice)
- Insurance authorization obtained
- Facility or service arranged
- Transfer paperwork completed
- Receiving facility contacted with warm handoff

☐ **Equipment and Medications**

- Durable medical equipment ordered
- Prescriptions sent to pharmacy
- Medication reconciliation completed
- Patient can access/afford medications

☐ **Follow-Up Appointments**

- Primary care appointment scheduled
- Specialist appointments arranged
- Transportation arranged
- Appointment information provided in writing

☐ **Community Resources**

- Referrals made for identified needs (food, housing, utilities, etc.)
- Contact information provided
- Warm handoffs completed when possible

☐ **Documentation**

- Discharge summary completed
- All interventions documented
- Barriers and solutions noted
- Receiving providers notified

☐ **Safety Planning**

- Home safety assessed
- Fall prevention addressed
- Emergency contacts identified
- Safety plan created if indicated (DV, suicide risk)

☐ **Patient Readiness**

- Patient understands plan
- Concerns addressed
- Questions answered
- Patient expresses readiness (or concerns documented)

# Glossary

**Advance directive:** Legal document outlining medical treatment preferences for situations where person cannot make decisions
**APS (Adult Protective Services):** State agency investigating abuse, neglect, or exploitation of vulnerable adults
**Capacity:** Clinical determination of person's ability to understand and make specific decisions
**Case management:** Coordinated services helping individuals access health and social services through planning and advocacy
**Comorbidity:** Presence of two or more medical conditions simultaneously
**CPS (Child Protective Services):** State agency investigating child abuse and neglect reports
**Cultural humility:** Ongoing process of self-reflection and learning about cultural differences with commitment to redressing power imbalances
**Discharge planning:** Process of preparing patient for transition from hospital to home or other setting
**DNR (Do Not Resuscitate):** Order indicating no CPR should be performed if cardiac or respiratory arrest occurs
**EMTALA:** Federal law requiring emergency departments to screen and stabilize anyone presenting, regardless of ability to pay
**HIPAA:** Federal law protecting privacy and security of health information
**Hospice:** Specialized care for terminally ill patients focusing on comfort and quality of life
**Informed consent:** Voluntary agreement to treatment based on understanding of risks, benefits, and alternatives
**Interdisciplinary team:** Professionals from different disciplines collaborating on patient care
**LCSW (licensed clinical social worker):** Advanced social work license permitting independent clinical practice
**LMSW (licensed master social worker):** Entry-level social work license requiring supervision for clinical practice
**Mandated reporter:** Professional required by law to report suspected abuse, neglect, or exploitation
**MPOA (medical power of attorney):** Legal document designating someone to make health care decisions
**Palliative care:** Specialized medical care for serious illness focused on symptom relief and quality of life
**POLST/MOLST:** Medical orders specifying life-sustaining treatment preferences for seriously ill patients
**Psychosocial assessment:** Clinical evaluation of psychological, social, spiritual, and environmental factors affecting health
**SBAR:** Structured communication framework (situation, background, assessment, recommendation)
**SDOH (social determinants of health):** Conditions in environments where people live, work, and age that affect health
**SNF (skilled nursing facility):** Licensed facility providing 24-hour nursing care and rehabilitation
**Structural racism:** Macro-level systems, policies, and practices that generate racial inequities
**Trauma-informed care:** Approach recognizing trauma's prevalence and impact, seeking to avoid retraumatization

# Recommended Reading


## Medical Social Work and Health Care Systems

Beder, J. (2006). *Hospital social work: The interface of medicine and caring*. Routledge.

Gehlert, S., & Browne, T. (Eds.). (2012). *Handbook of health social work* (2nd ed.). John Wiley & Sons.

## Ethics and Values

Beauchamp, T. L., & Childress, J. F. (2019). *Principles of biomedical ethics* (8th ed.). Oxford University Press.

Dolgoff, R., Harrington, D., & Loewenberg, F. M. (2012). *Ethical decisions for social work practice* (9th ed.). Brooks/Cole.

Reamer, F. G. (2013). *Social work values and ethics* (4th ed.). Columbia University Press.

## Cultural Competence and Social Justice

Baines, D. (Ed.). (2017). *Doing anti-oppressive practice: Social justice social work* (3rd ed.). Fernwood Publishing.

Sue, D. W., & Sue, D. (2016). *Counseling the culturally diverse: Theory and practice* (7th ed.). John Wiley & Sons.

## End-of-Life Care

Worden, J. W. (2018). *Grief counseling and grief therapy: A handbook for the mental health practitioner* (5th ed.). Springer Publishing Company.

## Professional Development

Kadushin, A., & Harkness, D. (2014). *Supervision in social work* (5th ed.). Columbia University Press.

Hepworth, D. H., et al. (2016). *Direct social work practice: Theory and skills* (10th ed.). Cengage Learning.

# Index

## A



## B



## C

## D



## E



## F



## G



## H

## I



## J



## L



## M

## T



## U



## V



## W

# About the Author

Dr. Kenshara Cravens-Knoxson is a Licensed Master Social Worker (LMSW), Licensed Graduate Social Worker (LGSW), and assistant professor at Prairie View A&M University. She earned her Ph.D. in social work from Walden University, with her dissertation titled "Experiences and Perceptions of Hospital Social Workers" exploring the complexities of medical social work practice.

Dr. Cravens-Knoxson brings extensive clinical experience to her teaching and scholarship, having worked in various healthcare settings including hospitals and managed care. Her practice expertise, combined with scholarly inquiry, positions her to bridge the gap between academic preparation and real-world healthcare practice.

As a first-generation college student, Dr. Cravens-Knoxson understands the transformative power of education and the challenges of navigating professional development. She is committed to empowering the next generation of social workers through excellence in teaching, mentorship, and scholarship that addresses the practical realities of healthcare social work.

Recognition for Dr. Cravens-Knoxson's work includes the Sages of Clinical Services Award (United Healthcare, 2021), "40 Under 40" recognition (Galveston Daily News), and Hometown Hero Award (Carolyn Taylor Lee Foundation). She founded Craving for A Change Foundation, Inc., a nonprofit focused on implementing social-emotional learning strategies for adolescent and young adult students in Galveston County public schools.

Dr. Cravens-Knoxson's professional mission centers on empowering others through service, mentorship, and compassion while advancing the social work profession's knowledge and impact in healthcare settings.